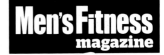

COMPLETE GUIDE TO
DUMB-BELL
TRAINING

By Jon Lipsey

Photography **Tom Miles**
Model **Matt Morgan@WAthletic**
Design **Ian Jackson**
Subeditor **Juliet Giles**

Equipment supplied by www.fitness-superstore.co.uk

Digital Production Manager **Nicky Baker**
Bookazine Manager **Dharmesh Mistry**
Operations Director **Robin Ryan**
Managing Director of Advertising
Julian Lloyd-Evans
Newstrade Director **David Barker**
Chief Operating Officer **Brett Reynolds**
Group Finance Director **Ian Leggett**
Chief Executive **James Tye**
Chairman **Felix Dennis**

MAGBOOK

The 'MagBook' brand is a trademark of Dennis Publishing Ltd,
30 Cleveland St, London W1T 4JD. Company registered in England.
All material © Dennis Publishing Ltd, licensed by Felden 2011,
and may not be reproduced in whole or part without the
consent of the publishers.

Complete Guide to Dumb-bell Training ISBN 1-907779-20-5

To license this product please contact Ornella Roccoletti on
+44 (0) 20 7907 6134 or email ornella_roccoletti@dennis.co.uk

reflex®

DIET PROTEIN

ARGUABLY THE MOST SOPHISTICATED PROTEIN BASED DIET SHAKE AVAILABLE TODAY BRINGING YOU THE LATEST ADVANCES IN NUTRACEUTICALS TO HELP CONTROL BODY WEIGHT AND FAT LEVELS.

PERFORMANCE

Diet Protein contains unique bioactive peptides & 100% RDA of calcium
Diet Protein uses a unique ratio of purified whey protein and micellar casein that may help curb appetite, boost glutathionine levels (antioxidants), promote healthy intestinal flora and provide essential amino acids for recovery from strenuous exercise. It also provides natural dairy calcium which is scientifically proven to assist in accelerating fat and weight loss by up to 25%.

Diet Protein contains Clarinol CLA, a safe, natural, research proven diet aid
One daily serving of Diet Protein provides 3.2g of Clarinol™ which has patents that allow them to claim; Clarinol™ reduces the amount of body fat, Clarinol™ reduces weight gain and Clarinol™ reduces the side effects from a low calorie diet. A recently completed six month clinical trial of Clarinol™ showed that the reduction in fat mass primarily occurs in the abdomen. Whilst other diet shakes might contain CLA it is often in smaller amounts. Research proves that you need to take 3.2g or more of CLA to see the best results.

HEALTH

Each serving of Diet Protein is packed with additional diet support. Green tea extract and L-carnitine L-tartrate are added given their long standing reputation for aiding dieters whilst Lactospore probiotics are added to promote general intestinal health.

Diet Protein contains no added sugar or maltodextrin. It's perfect for dieters wanting to restrict their carbohydrate content.

Diet Protein comes in a variety of mouthwatering flavours, all of which have been optimized by our taste testing panel to ensure that they are the best tasting diet shakes on the market.

PERFORMANCE & HEALTH WITHIN

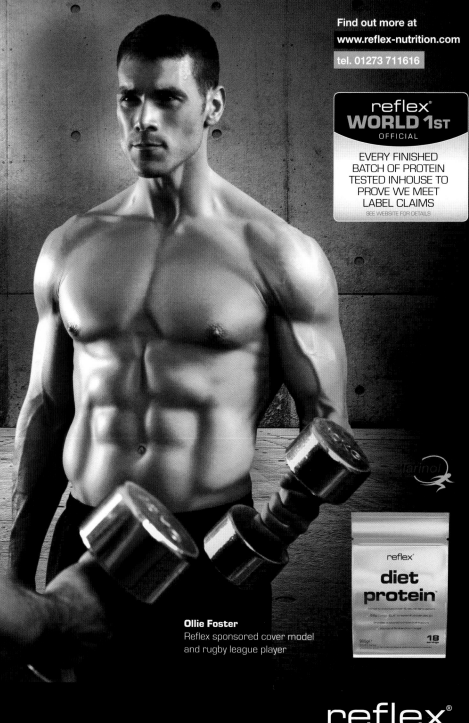

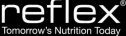

Foreword

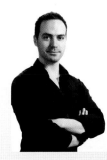

A lot of workout plans require you to make big changes to your life, such as giving up drinking for months. This guide is different, in that we only ask you to forgo a round of drinks. That's because the money you would have spent on that round should be invested in a set of dumb-bells. You see, for about £30 you can buy the most versatile and easy-to-master item of training kit available and start to build your best ever body.

What's in the guide

This guide tells you everything you need to know about training with dumb-bells, whether you're new to working out or you're a regular gym-goer. It starts with a chapter explaining the fundamentals of weight training. You then get 16 workout options for any training goal, whether you want to build a specific body part, such as your arms or chest, lose fat or get your workouts done as quickly as possible. There's also a three-month plan, involving three 40-minute workouts a week that will strip away fat and replace it with lean, hard muscle. The comprehensive form guides section will make sure you know how to execute every move and achieve your goals.

Jon Lipsey, Editor, Men's Fitness

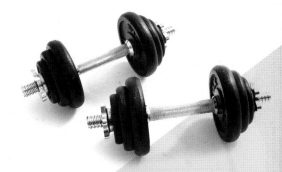

CONTENTS

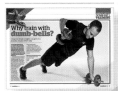
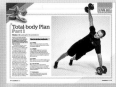
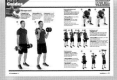

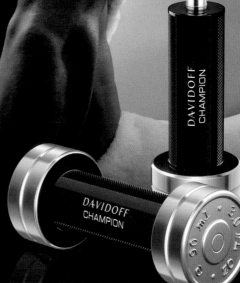

DAVIDOFF
CHAMPION

THE NEW MEN'S FRAGRANCE

Why train with dumb-bells?

Using these simple weights can give you fantastic results. Here's why

The humble dumb-bell is all you need to whip yourself into the shape of your life. Well, that's not strictly true because if you don't know how to use it effectively, then it's just a lump of metal. But with this guide you can make sure that lump of metal is transformed into a powerful fitness tool.

The advantages of training with dumb-bells are many: they're incredibly versatile; you can use them to target any muscle group; and – as well as a giving you a great-looking body – they improve a useful kind of fitness. Because when you hold one in each hand you have to completely control their movement, which ensures that each side of your body does an equal amount of work. They're also outstanding value, with a basic set costing as little as £30.

What's more you can use them for virtually any goal, whether you're aiming to increase your muscle size or trim your waistline. So, before you get started, here's the essential theory behind building muscle and burning fat.

Muscle growth fundamentals
You may think that to build muscle you need to shift huge weights every day but that's not the case. If you do an exercise with

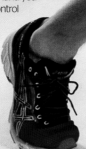

>

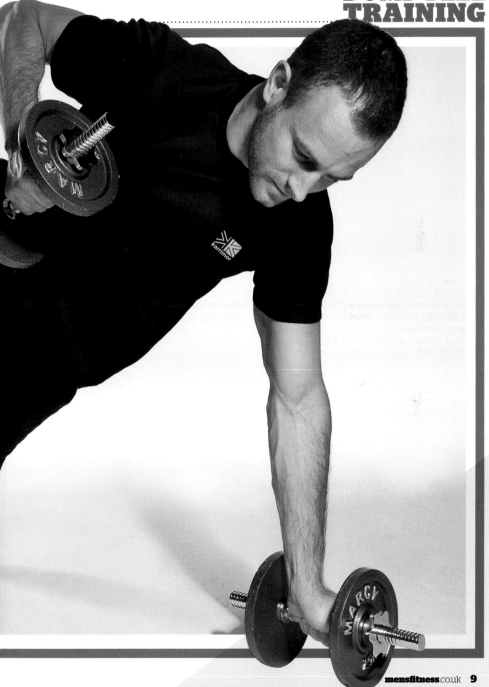

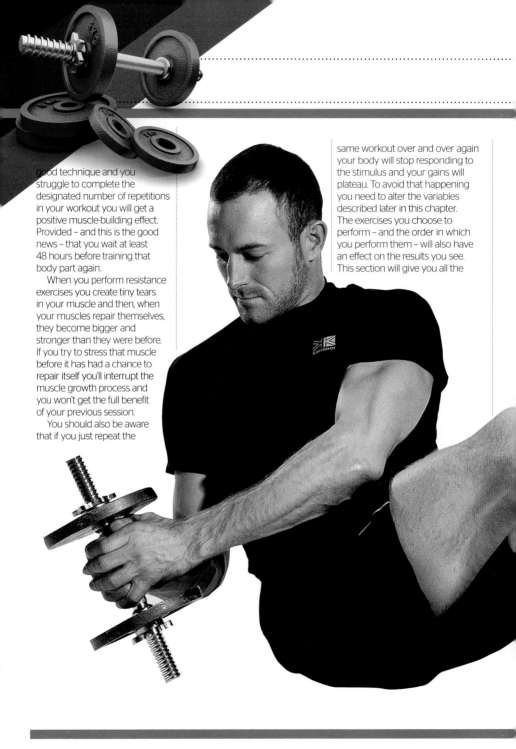

good technique and you struggle to complete the designated number of repetitions in your workout you will get a positive muscle-building effect. Provided – and this is the good news – that you wait at least 48 hours before training that body part again.

When you perform resistance exercises you create tiny tears in your muscle and then, when your muscles repair themselves, they become bigger and stronger than they were before. If you try to stress that muscle before it has had a chance to repair itself you'll interrupt the muscle growth process and you won't get the full benefit of your previous session.

You should also be aware that if you just repeat the same workout over and over again your body will stop responding to the stimulus and your gains will plateau. To avoid that happening you need to alter the variables described later in this chapter. The exercises you choose to perform – and the order in which you perform them – will also have an effect on the results you see. This section will give you all the information you need to decide what reps, sets, rest and tempo to use as well as a brief guide on how to order exercises.

Mastering fat loss

The subject of fat loss is one that's often misunderstood. Many people believe that if you want to ditch your spare tyre then you need to either do long, slow cardio sessions or cut out fat from your diet. The truth is, however, that lifting weights is the most effective route to fat loss.

Lifting weights is intense and demanding, which means

> 'If you just repeat the same workout over and over again your body will stop responding to the stimulus and your gains will plateau'

it creates an oxygen debt in your muscles that has to be replenished, all of which requires a lot of energy. As your body recovers from a session your fat stores are broken down and fatty acids are released into the blood and are used as fuel.

Also, your body will repair the damage you do to your muscles when you lift weights and this requires you to burn more calories. So going for a run may mean that you'll use extra calories for about 30 minutes after you finish but when you train with weights you'll burn extra calories for up to 48 hours after your session. Having a muscular physique will also help

you stay lean. Increased muscle mass is associated with a higher metabolic rate, so the more muscle you put on, the better your body will be at burning fat.

When you're lifting weights for fat loss, you need to keep your rest times between sets relatively short, to around 45 seconds. That will keep the intensity of your session high. And make sure that you lift to failure – the point at which you can't manage another rep with good form – on the final set of each exercise because that ensures that you damage your muscle fibres sufficiently to expend that extra energy.

>

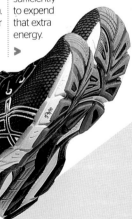

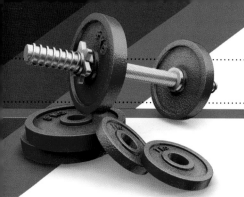

Workout variables

Starting a workout without knowing what you want to achieve, what exercises you're going to do or how you're going to perform them isn't going to give you optimum results. If you want to achieve your workout aims, you need to design – and stick to – a specific programme.

But you can't do that without understanding the key variables involved in how you perform each exercise and how you design your workouts. The main variables to think about are:

> **Repetitions**
Also known as reps, this is the number of times you lift a weight or perform a bodyweight exercise within a set.

> **Sets**
Groups of repetitions performed back to back.

> **Rest**
The inactive time you take between sets and exercises.

> **Tempo**
The speed at which reps are performed.

> **Frequency**
This refers to how often you perform a workout.

Repetitions

The number of repetitions you choose to perform will affect all the other variables and they have a huge impact on whether the primary effect of your workout is developing muscle strength, size or endurance.

Low reps, in the one to seven range, are best for building strength; eight to 12 reps is best for adding muscle mass; and 13-20 reps will develop muscle endurance. These are, however, on a spectrum rather than self-contained blocks. Performing three or seven repetitions of an exercise, for example, will have a strength-building effect but the seven repetitions will have more of a size development effect than performing three repetitions because it's closer to the size-gain range of the spectrum.

Sets

The number of sets you perform should be directly linked to the number of repetitions you do. Generally, the two should be inversely related so the more sets you do, the fewer reps you should perform and vice versa.

Studies show that the most effective length of a workout is around 45 minutes. After that, your training efforts can be counterproductive, because testosterone levels drop and stress hormone levels rise. So, if you include a high number of exercises in your workout you may need to reduce the number sets.

If you're very new to training, you may want to consider doing one or two sets of each exercise to get your muscles used to the movements without overstressing them. As you improve, you can increase the total number of sets.

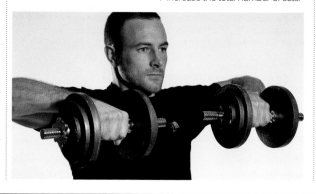

'If you want to achieve your workout aims, you need to design – and stick to – a specific programme'

Tempo

The speed at which you complete each phase of a rep also plays a part in the training effect you get from the lift. Doing ten repetitions of a biceps curl as fast as possible won't have the same effect on your muscles as doing the move slowly.

To maximise strength and size gains, conditioning research suggests that your muscles should be under tension for between 40 to 70 seconds each set, provided you're not using extremely low repetition ranges. Lifting in this way will cause you to use anaerobic energy, which produces lactate and prompts the release of testosterone and growth hormones.

It's also important to use the right lifting speed within a rep. To make sure your muscles are under tension for long enough, take one second to lift the weight, pause then take three seconds to lower it. The reason you should take longer to lower the weight is that size gains are best made during the eccentric (lowering) phase of the lift.

Some exercises, however, such as the snatch, have to be performed at speed because they require explosive movements to lift a weight that's heavy enough for you to get a training benefit.

Rest

The rest you take determines whether or not you're able to complete the next section of your workout. As a rule, sets with few reps will require more rest, as they train the nervous system and fast-twitch muscle fibres, which fatigue easily and take longer to recover. As you increase the number of reps you train your slow-twitch fibres, which are harder to fatigue.

Those new to weight training may need to take longer rests than more experienced lifters, who have a higher tolerance to the lactate produced during lifts. How much you weigh can also affect your rest times, with heavier lifters needing longer to recover between sets.

Your rest periods are effective when you can reach positive failure on the last rep of the set. This means you are unable to lift the weight with perfect form but are able to lower it under control. If you don't reach that point by the end of your set, your rest periods may be too long. ➤

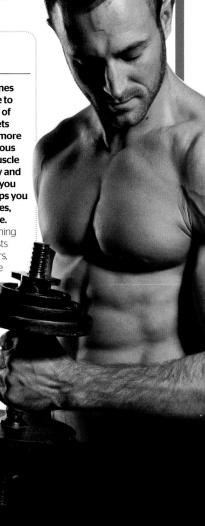

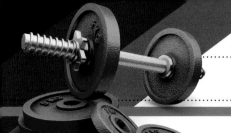

Selecting and ordering exercises

The exercises you should perform depend on what you want to achieve. The sample workouts in the next chapter will give you an example of how to select exercises according to goals such as developing a particular body part, losing fat or increasing explosive power.

Structuring your workout properly is important because different exercises place different demands on your body. The following guidelines will help you to structure your workouts to maximise muscle growth and strength gains while also minimising your injury risk.

Do big explosive moves early in your workout
Explosive exercises, such as the jump squat, are very demanding so they need to be performed when you are relatively fresh. Do these moves early on in your workout and before simpler moves, such as triceps extensions.

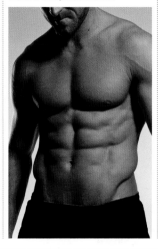

Do difficult moves first and easier moves last
Complete large muscle group moves, such as squats, at the beginning of your workout to make sure you keep perfect form and your core is strong enough to stabilise your body. Easier moves, such as biceps curls, should be done later in the workout.

Save core moves until last
Similarly, if you perform the moves designed to strengthen your core muscles too early on in your workout you'll fatigue these muscles. Then, when you come to do big dynamic lifts, such as lunges that call on your core muscles to stabilise your movement, these muscles may not be able to provide adequate support for the move. As well as losing form you'll also increase your risk of injury.

Frequency

How many workouts you do each week is likely to be influenced by work and family commitments. The good news, if you do lead a busy life, is that you don't need to work out seven days a week to see great results. Doing between three and five workouts a week should be sufficient to achieve your workout goals.

Exactly how many sessions you do depends on a number of factors. One thing that should influence training frequency is what sort of workouts you're doing. A hard full-body session may mean that you need to leave at least 48 hours between sessions in order for your muscles to recover and repair themselves to be stronger than before. If you're focussing on a particular body part each workout, you may be able to train the following day if you work on a different body part.

One common mistake is to think that the more workouts you do, the stronger and more muscular you'll become. In fact it's while you're resting, and not while you're working out, that your muscles get bigger and stronger. If you stress your muscles before they've had a chance to repair themselves this may cause overtraining, where you lose strength and muscle mass and feel lethargic.

Some muscle groups take longer to recover than others. Larger muscle groups, particularly those with a comparatively higher percentage of fast-twitch muscle fibres, such as the hamstrings may take longer to recover than some smaller muscle groups, such as the calves.

Know your
muscles

There are more than 600 muscles in the body. These are the key ones you'll be targeting during your workouts

Jargon buster
Concentric contraction
This is a controlled shortening of your muscle, such as the upwards phase of a biceps curl.

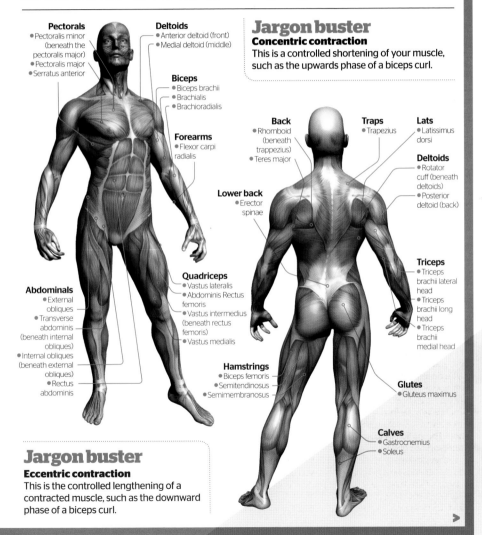

Pectorals
- Pectoralis minor (beneath the pectoralis major)
- Pectoralis major
- Serratus anterior

Deltoids
- Anterior deltoid (front)
- Medial deltoid (middle)

Biceps
- Biceps brachii
- Brachialis
- Brachioradialis

Forearms
- Flexor carpi radialis

Abdominals
- External obliques
- Transverse abdominis (beneath internal obliques)
- Internal obliques (beneath external obliques)
- Rectus abdominis

Quadriceps
- Vastus lateralis
- Abdominis Rectus femoris
- Vastus intermedius (beneath rectus femoris)
- Vastus medialis

Back
- Rhomboid (beneath trappezius)
- Teres major

Lower back
- Erector spinae

Traps
- Trapezius

Lats
- Latissimus dorsi

Deltoids
- Rotator cuff (beneath deltoids)
- Posterior deltoid (back)

Triceps
- Triceps brachii lateral head
- Triceps brachii long head
- Triceps brachii medial head

Hamstrings
- Biceps femoris
- Semitendinosus
- Semimembranosus

Glutes
- Gluteus maximus

Calves
- Gastrocnemius
- Soleus

Jargon buster
Eccentric contraction
This is the controlled lengthening of a contracted muscle, such as the downward phase of a biceps curl.

Dumb-bell
buyer's guide

Chose the weights that suit your needs

Fixed dumb-bells

As the name implies, the weight on these dumb-bells can't be altered. You can either buy them individually or as part of a set that increases in weight at regular increments. It's quick and easy to find your desired weight but the downside is that they're relatively expensive and they take up a lot of space, which is why you're more likely to find a set in the gym than in a home training set-up. If you do invest in a set, it's a good idea to get ones with hexagonal shaped ends because they can be used on the floor for exercises such as renegade rows and T press-ups without rolling around.

Adjustable dumb-bells

This type of dumb-bell lets you change the weight you lift without having to mess around with weight plates. The most sophisticated versions allow you to position a dial next to the value of the weight you want to lift. When you then lift the dumb-bell bar, part of the weight is left behind, leaving you with exactly the amount of weight you want to lift. They are more expensive than the plate-loaded dumb-bells but they are more convenient and allow you to stick rigidly to rest periods.

Plate-loaded dumb-bells

These are the low-cost option, so a good choice if you're on a tight budget. They have two collars that secure plates of different increments to both ends of the dumb-bell bar. Once loaded they work your body in exactly the same way as fixed and adjustable dumb-bells. The only downside is that it can be time consuming to keep altering the weights between exercises.

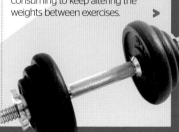

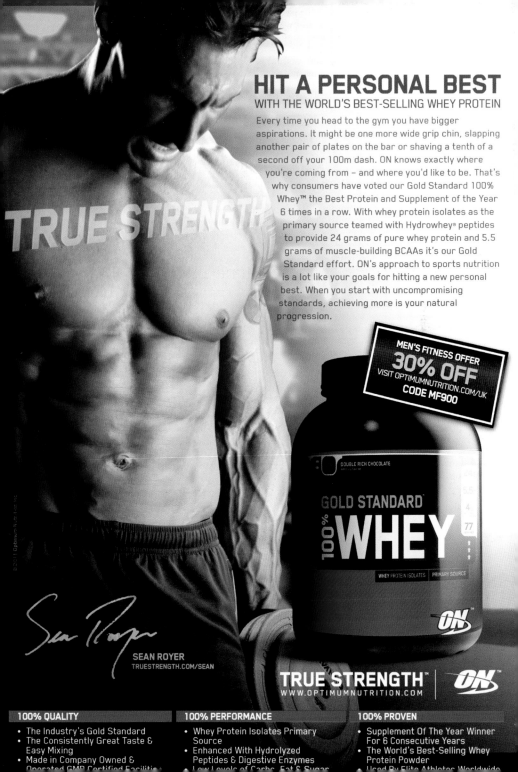

HIT A PERSONAL BEST
WITH THE WORLD'S BEST-SELLING WHEY PROTEIN

Every time you head to the gym you have bigger aspirations. It might be one more wide grip chin, slapping another pair of plates on the bar or shaving a tenth of a second off your 100m dash. ON knows exactly where you're coming from – and where you'd like to be. That's why consumers have voted our Gold Standard 100% Whey™ the Best Protein and Supplement of the Year 6 times in a row. With whey protein isolates as the primary source teamed with Hydrowhey® peptides to provide 24 grams of pure whey protein and 5.5 grams of muscle-building BCAAs it's our Gold Standard effort. ON's approach to sports nutrition is a lot like your goals for hitting a new personal best. When you start with uncompromising standards, achieving more is your natural progression.

DOUBLE RICH CHOCOLATE

GOLD STANDARD
100% WHEY

WHEY PROTEIN ISOLATES | PRIMARY SOURCE

SEAN ROYER
TRUESTRENGTH.COM/SEAN

TRUE STRENGTH™
WWW.OPTIMUMNUTRITION.COM

ON™

100% QUALITY
- The Industry's Gold Standard
- The Consistently Great Taste & Easy Mixing
- Made in Company Owned & Operated GMP Certified Facilitie

100% PERFORMANCE
- Whey Protein Isolates Primary Source
- Enhanced With Hydrolyzed Peptides & Digestive Enzymes
- Low Levels of Carbs, Fat & Sugar

100% PROVEN
- Supplement Of The Year Winner For 6 Consecutive Years
- The World's Best-Selling Whey Protein Powder
- Used By Elite Athletes Worldwide

Pre-workout
warm-up

Get your body primed and ready for muscle growth with this quick pre-workout warm-up

The warm-up is the part of a workout most men are likely to overlook. It may seem a bit dull but the benefits make it worth doing. The purpose of a warm-up is simple: to raise your core temperature and prepare your muscles for the work to come.

Dynamic stretches (described below) will target the muscles you're going to use during the workout so they're ready for lifting. Dynamic stretches involve moving continuously, placing the muscle under

tension a little bit more with each repetition, which prepares your muscle joints and nerves for the actions they're about to perform. They differ from static stretches (see pages 20-21), which, according to the latest exercise science research, should not be done before a workout. A study published in *The Journal Of Strength And Conditioning Research* found that pre-workout static stretches reduce the power available to a muscle during the workout.

Warm-up dynamic stretches

Do ten repetitions of each of the following stretches, alternating sides with each rep where appropriate. Start gently and aim to increase the range of motion with each rep.

» Lunge with reverse flye
- Step forward and bend your knees
- Spread your arms wide

» Squat to reach
- Squat down with your back straight
- Stand up and raise your arms

» Woodchop
- Start in a squat with your arms outside your thigh
- Bring your arms up and across your body as you rise up

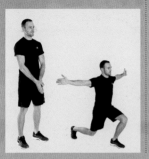
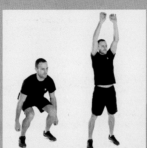
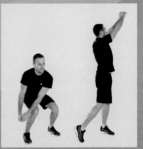

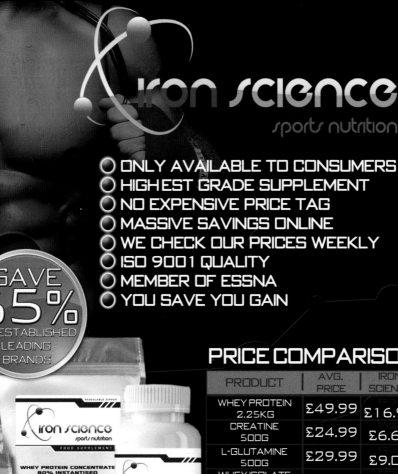

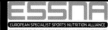

Post-workout
warm-down

Do the following stretches after a weights session to increase your flexibility and speed up your recovery

After you've finished your workout spend five minutes doing some gentle cardio, such as jogging on the spot, to bring your heart rate down. Then perform the following stretches, paying particular attention to those that target the muscles you worked during your session.

Get into the stretch position and allow your muscle to relax. As you place pressure on your muscle you should be able to feel it relaxing and lengthening. You can slowly increase the pressure on the muscle throughout the duration of the stretch but you should never force or 'bounce' it because that can damage the muscle. Hold each stretch for between 15 and 30 seconds but if you feel any pain, stop immediately.

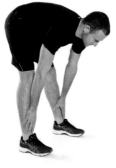

> Hamstrings
Keep your legs straight and lean forward to feel the stretch in your hamstrings.

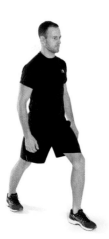

> Calves
Take a step forward and press your back heel down to feel the stretch in your rear calf.

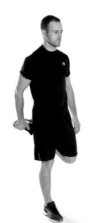

> Quads
Hold your ankle and push your hips forward to feel the stretch in your thigh.

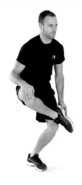

> Glutes
Stand on one leg and balance the bottom of your raised shin on your standing knee. Sink down until you feel the stretch in your glutes.

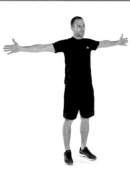

> Chest
With your palms facing forwards, take your arms back to feel the stretch across your chest.

> Abs
Lie on the floor with your palms directly below your shoulders and your elbows tucked in. Then raise your shoulders while keeping your hips on the ground.

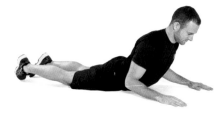

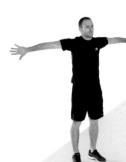

> Triceps
Bend one arm at the elbow and drop it down behind your back. With your other arm, push down gently on your elbow.

> Lats
Kneel down and extend one arm out so it rests on the ground. Press down on your leading arm to feel the stretch down your side.

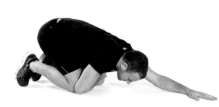

> Biceps
With your palms facing backwards, press your arms behind you to feel the stretch in your biceps.

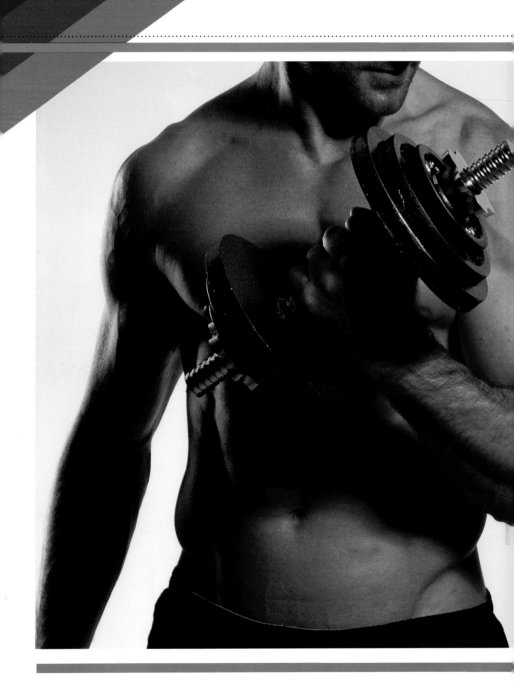

Dumb-bell
Workouts

This section contains workouts that will
help you achieve any exercise goal >

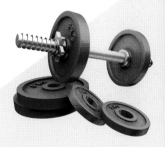

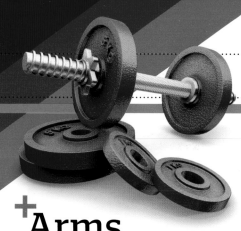

- **Do exercises 1-6 in order**
- **Rest for 1 minute between sets**
- **Rest for 2 minutes between exercises**

1

Diamond press-up
> **Sets** 3 > **Reps** 10

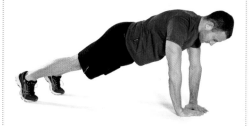

⁺Arms
Workout

WHY DO IT?

Build arms that fill your T-shirts

The fastest way to build big arms isn't to crank out as many biceps curls as you can. True, that type of move is included in this workout, but it's only one part of the puzzle.

To increase the size and strength of your arms you need to work your biceps from a variety of different angles. The concentration curl isolates your biceps and allows you to lift a heavy weight. The hammer curl changes your grip and challenges your forearms. The final biceps move, the Zottman curl targets your biceps in the lifting phase and your forearms in the lowering phase.

Between biceps moves you perform three triceps moves. These are crucial because they allow your biceps to recover and they also build strength and size on the backs of your upper arms. In fact, your triceps make up two thirds of your upper arm mass, so working those muscles will provide you with quick T-shirt-filling gains.

> **Form guide** p105

4

Hammer curl
> **Sets** 3 > **Reps** 10

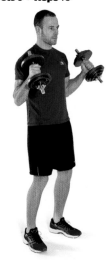

> **Form guide** p84

FIT TIP > To make your arm moves even more effective, make sure you really squeeze the muscle at the top of the move, such as the up phase of a biceps curl.

2 Concentration curl
> **Sets** 2 > **Reps** 10 each side

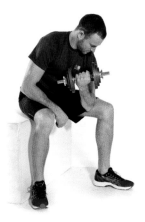

> **Form guide** p83

3 Two-arm kickback
> **Sets** 3 > **Reps** 10

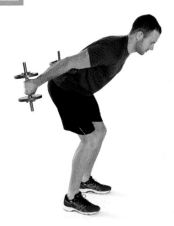

> **Form guide** p87

5 Zottman curl
> **Sets** 3 > **Reps** 10

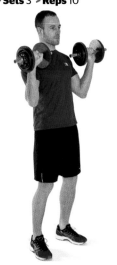

> **Form guide** p83

6 Overhead triceps extension
> **Sets** 2
> **Reps** 10 each side

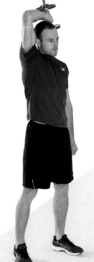

> **Form guide** p86

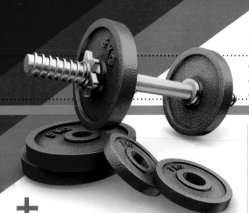

Do this ↘

- **Do exercises 1-6 in order**
- **Rest for 1 minute between sets**
- **Rest for 2 minutes between exercises**

⁺Chest & back
Workout

WHY DO IT?

Get a strong-looking upper body

Most men are far more concerned with building a big chest than they are with developing a strong back. That's the wrong approach for two reasons. By focusing on your chest at the expense of your back you'll develop poor posture and a hunched-over appearance. You'll also be missing out on an aesthetic V-shaped torso, which you get by working on the lats muscles of your back.

This workout contains three chest moves and three back moves and you alternate between the two body parts. The first two moves will also work your core because the muscles around your spine have to work hard to keep your body stable. The second back move, the shrug, targets your upper back while the second chest move allows you to lift heavy weights because you're doing the move from a stable position. The reverse flye really isolates your back muscles while the dumb-bell jab is an explosive way to end the workout.

FIT TIP >
Bent-over rows put more stress on your lower back than most back moves, according to the *Journal of Strength & Conditioning Research*, so make sure you engage your spine when doing the move.

 Bent-over row
> **Sets** 3 > **Reps** 10

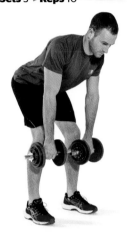

> **Form guide** p94

 Floor press
> **Sets** 3 > **Reps** 10

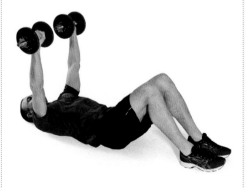

> **Form guide** p102

2 Dumb-bell press-up
> **Sets** 3 > **Reps** 10

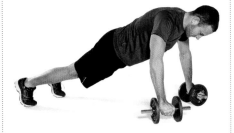
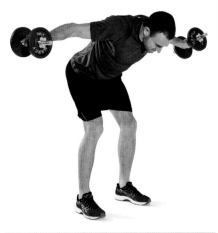

> **Form guide** p100

3 Shrug
> **Sets** 3
> **Reps** 10

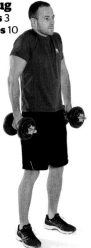

> **Form guide** p97

5 Bent-over flye
> **Sets** 3 > **Reps** 10

> **Form guide** p98

6 Punch
> **Sets** 2 > **Reps** 10 each side

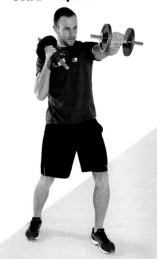

> **Form guide** p103

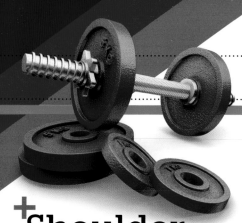

Do this ↘

- **Do exercises 1-6 in order**
- **Rest for 1 minute between sets**
- **Rest for 2 minutes between exercises**

+Shoulder
Workout

WHY DO IT?

Build broad boulder shoulders

Your shoulders require special attention, which is why we've devised this workout. The big muscles in the joint have the capacity to shift a large amount of weight but if the small stabilising muscles that are deep in the joint are ignored you could end up with an injury that's hard to heal.

This workout begins with two exercises – external and internal rotations – that strengthen the deep lying stabilising muscles. They will also warm-up your joint for the bigger lifts, such as the seated shoulder press, that follow. As with any body part, it's important to work the shoulders from a variety of angles. The lateral raise will target your middle shoulders, the front raise targets your front shoulders and the halo targets the front, middle and rear shoulder.

FIT TIP **>** One recent US study found that 36 per cent of resistance training injuries are shoulder related. The top two causes were muscle imbalance and poor technique but doing the one-sided moves in this workout with proper form will help you stay injury free.

1 External rotations
> Sets 2 **> Reps** 12-15 each side

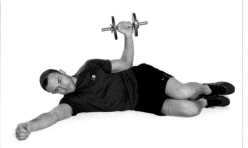

> Form guide p123

4 Lateral raise
> Sets 3 **> Reps** 10

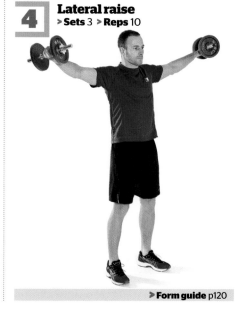

> Form guide p120

Internal rotations
> **Sets** 2 > **Reps** 12-15 each side

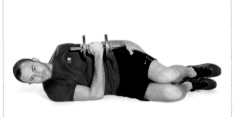

> **Form guide** p123

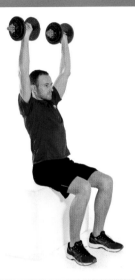

Seated shoulder press
> **Sets** 3
> **Reps** 10

> **Form guide** p118

Front raise
> **Sets** 3 > **Reps** 10

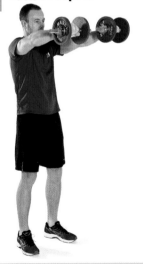

> **Form guide** p121

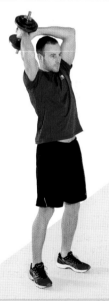

Halo
> **Sets** 3
> **Reps** 10

> **Form guide** p124

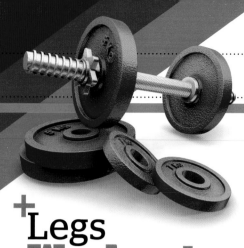

Do this ⬂

- **Do exercises 1-5 in order**
- **Rest for 1 minute between sets**
- **Rest for 2 minutes between exercises**

+Legs
Workout

WHY DO IT?

Get a balanced, powerful physique

Gyms are full of men who devote all their training time to their upper body and none to their legs. Aside from giving themselves an odd looking physique they are missing a training trick because leg moves, such as squats and lunges, target the big muscles of your glutes, quads and hamstrings, and working these areas hits a huge number of muscle fibres, which floods your body with growth hormones.

Strong legs will also improve your performance in sports – particularly explosive power sports such as rugby – but to work them effectively you need to use a variety of exercises. The first move in this workout works the quads while the second targets your hamstrings. The reverse lunge is great for developing balance and co-ordination because we are generally not used to moving backwards while controlling a weight. Finally, the side step-up gets you moving in a different plane of motion and is great at developing those frequently overlooked glute muscles.

FIT TIP > If you find the reverse lunge difficult, start by taking a step backwards, pausing then lowering into the lunge. Then you can work up to one fluid movement.

1 **Bulgarian split squat**
> **Sets** 2 > **Reps** 10 each side

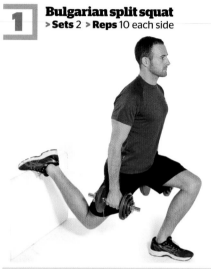

> **Form guide** p114

4 **Reverse lunge**
> **Sets** 2 > **Reps** 10 each side

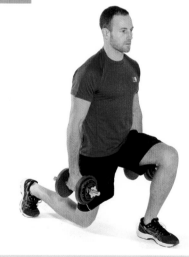

> **Form guide** p113

2
One-leg Romanian deadlift
> **Sets** 2 > **Reps** 10 each side

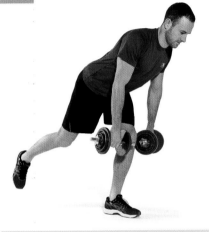

> **Form guide** p111

3

Sumo squat
> **Sets** 3
> **Reps** 10

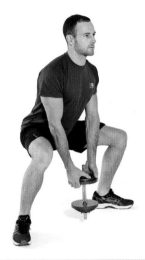

> **Form guide** p107

5
Side step-up
> **Sets** 2 > **Reps** 10 each side

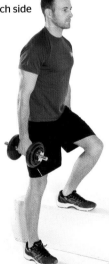

> **Form guide** p116

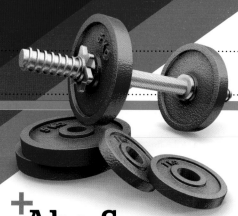

+Abs & core
Workout

Do this ↘

- **Do exercises 1-6 in order**
- **Rest for 1 minute between sets**
- **Rest for 2 minutes between exercises**

WHY DO IT?

Build a rock-solid six-pack

You won't be able to build strong abdominal muscles and a solid core simply by doing thousands of sit-ups. You need to target all the muscles of your midsection, and that means doing exercises that work your upper, lower and side abs as well as your deep lying muscles.

The first move in this workout involves moving the weight from a high to low position while simultaneously moving it from one side of your body to the other. This teaches your upper and lower body to work together to control the dumb-bell across a big range of motion. The side plank snatch also requires good core control as you balance in an unstable position while doing a complicated dumb-bell movement.

The other moves in the workout make sure that you work every area of your abs – including those hard to hit, and frequently overlooked, lower abdominals.

1 | **Woodchop**
> **Sets** 2 > **Reps** 10 each side

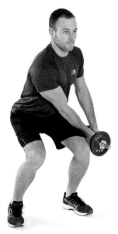

> **Form guide** p128

4 | **Dumb-bell side bend**
> **Sets** 2
> **Reps** 10 each side

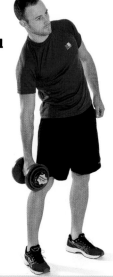

> **Form guide** p92

FIT TIP > Try to maintain a good posture throughout the day, even while sitting at your desk, as that will instill good habits for your deep-lying stabilising muscles.

2 Side plank snatch
> **Sets** 2 > **Reps** 10 each side

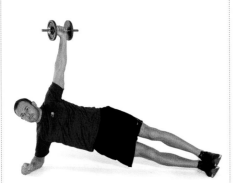

> **Form guide** p91

3 Rollout
> **Sets** 3 > **Reps** 10

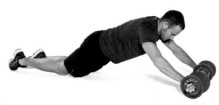

> **Form guide** p93

5 Weighted hip raise
> **Sets** 3
> **Reps** 10

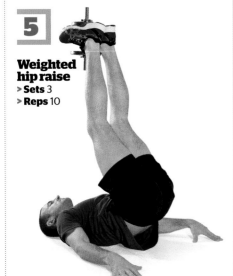

> **Form guide** p90

6 Side plank with lateral raise
> **Sets** 2 > **Reps** 10 each side

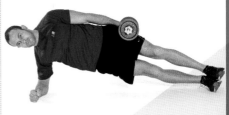

> **Form guide** p91

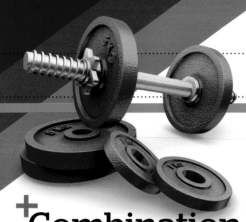

Do this ↘

- **Do exercises 1-4 in order**
- **Rest for 1 minute between sets**
- **Rest for 2 minutes between exercises**

+Combination Moves

WHY DO IT?

Save time and burn calories

This four-move workout may look easy, but in fact it's among the most challenging in this book. That's because the exercises are combination moves – two or more exercises spliced together to create one big move. They may be difficult but they're an excellent way of engaging your brain with what you're doing.

The big ranges of motion mean that this workout will burn loads of calories, and the high-intensity nature of the session also means that you'll continue burning calories long after you've stopped exercising because your body has to make a huge effort to recover.

One advantage of this type of move is that you can work more than one plane of motion in the same move. This teaches your body to work as a unit, improving your co-ordination. The final move in the session, the Turkish get-up, isn't technically a combination move but it's such a useful full-body move that it gives you the same sort of benefits as the other three exercises.

FIT TIP > Because all of the moves in this workout are full-body moves that require high amounts of balance and co-ordination, leave your ego at the door and keep the weights light.

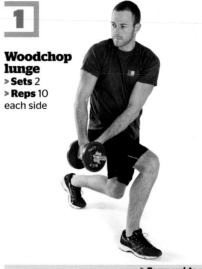

1

Woodchop lunge
> **Sets** 2
> **Reps** 10 each side

> **Form guide** p129

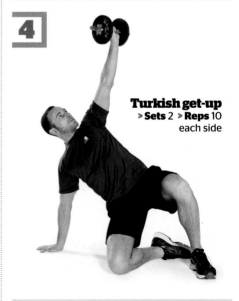

4

Turkish get-up
> **Sets** 2 > **Reps** 10 each side

> **Form guide** p127

2 | **Romanian deadlift to row**
> **Sets** 3 > **Reps** 10

3 | **Squat to curl to press**
> **Sets** 3 > **Reps** 10

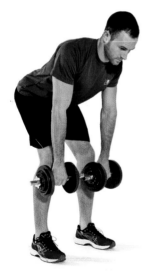

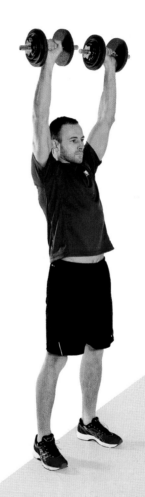

 > Form guide p111

> Form guide p108

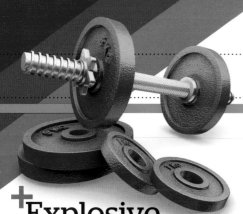

Do this ↘

- **Do exercises 1-5 in order**
- **Rest for 1 minute between sets**
- **Rest for 2 minutes between exercises**

+Explosive power
Workout

WHY DO IT?

Build strength for the sports field

If you want to train to be better at sport, you need to use moves that work your body in a way that's similar to the type of movements you make on the sportsfield. That's why doing slow tempo moves isn't appropriate, unless you play your sport in slow motion.

It's also important to select moves that involve large ranges of movement and ones that require your upper and lower body to work together. The 180-degree rotating woodchop, for example, calls on your upper and lower body to work together while also requiring good core strength to control the rotational movement.

The other moves are all power variations of conventional exercises. Doing a ballistic press-up will give you great pushing power, which is useful for sports such as rugby. Doing a jump squat, rather than a conventional squat, will recruit your fast-twitch muscle fibres, which are associated with explosive movements such as sprinting.

FIT TIP > Explosive workouts are particularly demanding so don't use this training method more than once a week and give yourself two days to recover before your next session.

1 | 180° rotating woodchop
> **Sets** 4 > **Reps** 6 each side

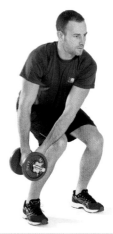

> **Form guide** p129

4 | Push press
> **Sets** 4 > **Reps** 8

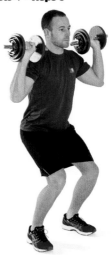

> **Form guide** p119

2 Ballistic press-up
> **Sets** 5 > **Reps** 5

> **Form guide** p105

3 Jump squat
> **Sets** 4 > **Reps** 8

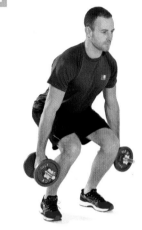

> **Form guide** p107

5 Punch
> **Sets** 2 > **Reps** 10 each side

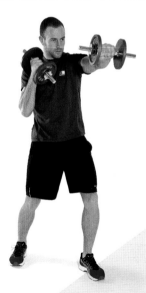

> **Form guide** p89

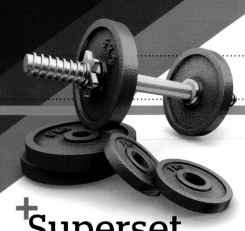

Do this ↘

- **Do 3 supersets for each group**
- **Rest for 60 seconds between supersets**
- **Rest for 90 seconds between superset groups**

1a **Floor press**
> **Sets** 3 > **Reps** 10

⁺Superset
Workout

WHY DO IT?

Great calorie burn and fat loss effect

A superset is any two exercises performed back to back without rest, but the most common type are antagonistic supersets. This means that you work opposing muscle groups, such as your chest and back, which in turn means that while you work one muscle group the other has a chance to recover. This way you get balanced muscle growth because you're not favouring your chest over your back, for example, which would give you a hunched posture.

Other ways of supersetting include performing two exercises that target the same muscle group or two completely unrelated muscle groups.

A further benefit of supersets is that you will reduce the amount of time you spend doing your workout because you slash your rest periods. That also means that you keep the intensity of your session high, which allows you to torch calories. In one recent study, those who used supersets expended nearly 50 per cent more energy than a group who used simple sets.

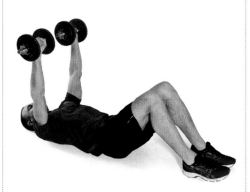

> **Form guide** p102

1b **Upright row**
> **Sets** 3 > **Reps** 10

FIT TIP > You can create your own supersets by pairing two exercises that work opposing muscle groups such as your chest and back, biceps and triceps and quads and hamstrings.

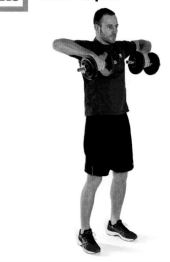

> **Form guide** p96

Bulgarian split squat
> **Sets** 2 > **Reps** 10 each side

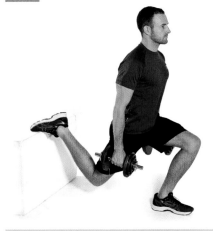

> **Form guide** p114

Romanian deadlift
> **Sets** 2 > **Reps** 12

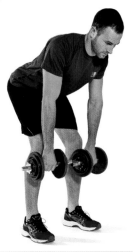

> **Form guide** p110

Biceps curl
> **Sets** 2
> **Reps** 10 each side

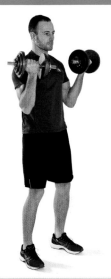

> **Form guide** p82

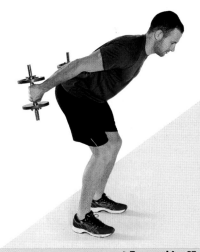

Two-arm kickback
> **Sets** 2 > **Reps** 12

> **Form guide** p87

Do this ↘

- **Do exercises 1-6 in order**
- **Rest for 1 minute between sets**
- **Rest for 2 minutes between exercises**

+Unilateral Workout

WHY DO IT?

Get balanced muscle growth

Almost everyone is stronger in one side of their body than the other, which is why you need to do unilateral moves that work one side of your body at a time. Dumb-bells are particularly good for unilateral workouts because you're controlling the same weight with each side. That's not the case when you use a barbell, for example, because your stronger side will naturally try to take more of the strain.

Any move that involves two dumb-bells is going to give you balanced muscle growth but you can really make sure that you get even muscle development by doing moves that alternate between sides of the body.

FIT TIP > If you can't lift as much weight with your weaker side as you can with your strong side, don't lower the weight. Use the same weight and do as many reps as you can until you reach failure.

1

Alternating hammer curl with twist
> **Sets** 2
> **Reps** 10 each side

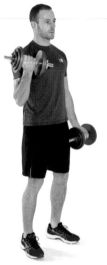

> **Form guide** p84

4

Dumb-bell hook
> **Sets** 2 > **Reps** 10 each side

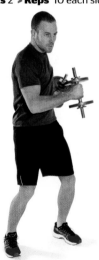

> **Form guide** p103

2

Rotating squat press
> **Sets** 2
> **Reps** 10
each side

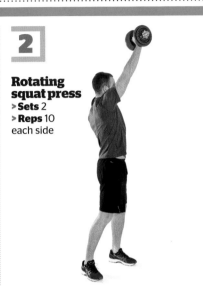

> **Form guide** p109

Step-up
Sets 2
> **Reps** 10
each side

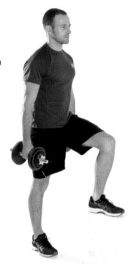

> **Form guide** p116

5

Front/lateral raise
> **Sets** 2 > **Reps** 10 each side

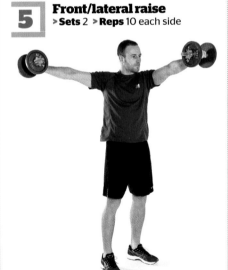

> **Form guide** p121

Saxon side bend
> **Sets** 2
> **Reps** 10
each side

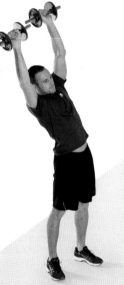

> **Form guide** p92

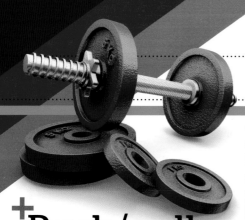

⁺Push/pull **Workout**

WHY DO IT?

Improve posture and get balanced muscle growth

In a push/pull workout you do the same number of moves that are classed as a pushing movement as you do exercises that are classed as pulling movements. A pushing exercise is anything that works either your chest, shoulders, quads, triceps or calves while a pulling movement will target your back, hamstrings, biceps or abs.

This workout alternates between pushing and pulling movements but you can do an entire workout devoted to either pushing or pulling movements, provided you do another workout involving the other movement in your next session.

FIT TIP > If you alternate between push and pull moves you can turn your session into a superset workout (see p38) by pairing moves and adjusting your rest times.

Do this ↘

- Do exercises 1-6 in order
- Rest for 1 minute between sets
- Rest for 2 minutes between exercises

1 T press-up
> **Sets** 2 > **Reps** 8 each side

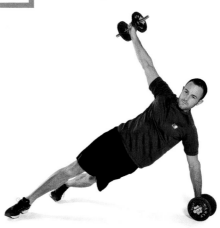

> **Form guide** p101

4 Upright row to shrug
> **Sets** 3
> **Reps** 10

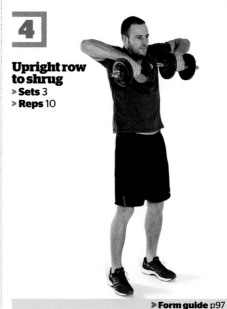

> **Form guide** p97

2 One-leg Romanian deadlift
> **Sets** 2 > **Reps** 10 each side

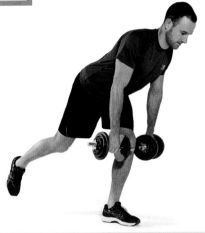

> **Form guide** p111

3 Arnold press
> **Sets** 3
> **Reps** 10

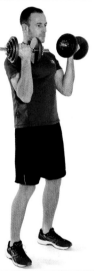

> **Form guide** p119

5 Overhead triceps extension
> **Sets** 2
> **Reps** 10 each side

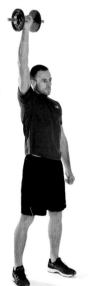

> **Form guide** p86

6 Hammer curl
> **Sets** 3
> **Reps** 10

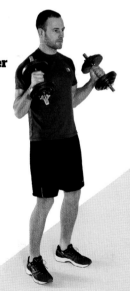

> **Form guide** p84

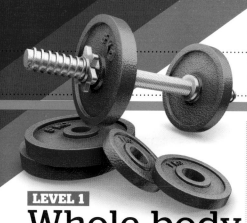

Do this ↘

- Do exercises 1-6 in order
- Rest for 1 minute between sets
- Rest for 2 minutes between exercises

Squat to curl to press
> **Sets** 3
> **Reps** 10

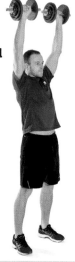

> **Form guide** p108

LEVEL 1

Whole-body Workout

WHY DO IT?

Build a strong and stable body

This workout is suitable for beginners but it can also be used by experienced weight trainers. The difference is that beginners should start with a light weight and build up. Whole body training is particularly suitable for beginners because no single body part is overly stressed. By working every part of your body you achieve all-over muscle growth.

It's important to include compound moves (exercises that target more than one muscle group) even at an entry level because this will teach your body to work as a unit. It will also promote good movement patterns and balance, which you'll need when you move on to levels two and three, which involve more difficult exercises.

Lunge
> **Sets** 2   > **Reps** 10 each side

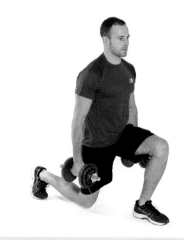

> **Form guide** p112

FIT TIP > The most important thing in this workout is to get used to performing good movement patterns in key exercises such as the squat to curl to press and the lunge.

2 Press-up
> **Sets** 3 > **Reps** 10

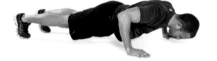

> **Form guide** p104

3 Reverse-grip bent-over row
> **Sets** 3 > **Reps** 10

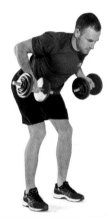

> **Form guide** p95

5 Alternating shoulder press
> **Sets** 2
> **Reps** 10 each side

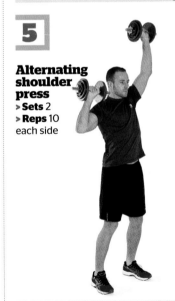

> **Form guide** p118

6 Crunch
> **Sets** 3 > **Reps** 10

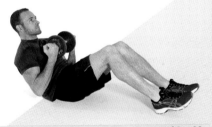

> **Form guide** p88

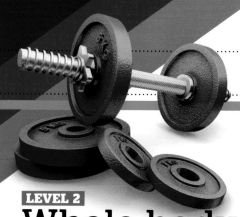

Do this ↘

- **Do exercises 1-6 in order**
- **Rest for 1 minute between sets**
- **Rest for 2 minutes between exercises**

LEVEL 2

Whole-body Workout

WHY DO IT?

Challenge yourself to build an impressive physique

The exercises get noticeably harder in level two than they were in level one. If you've already done the level one workout you'll have established good movement patterns in key exercises such as squats and press-ups.

In this workout you're still working similar movements but each one is more difficult. Doing a diamond press-up, for example, is harder than a standard press-up because it places much more emphasis on your triceps.

Bulgarian split squat
> **Sets** 2 > **Reps** 10 each side

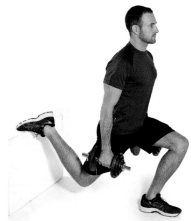

> **Form guide** p114

One-leg Romanian deadlift
> **Sets** 2 > **Reps** 10 each side

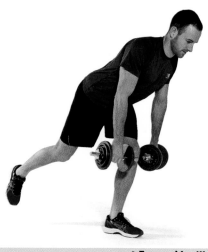

> **Form guide** p111

FIT TIP > If you struggle to complete the number of reps for any exercise, don't compromise your form. Simply do as many reps as you can with perfect form then move on to the next move.

2 Diamond press-up
> **Sets** 3 > **Reps** 10

> **Form guide** p105

3 Renegade row
> **Sets** 3 > **Reps** 10

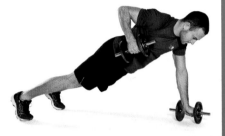

> **Form guide** p99

5 Curl to press
> **Sets** 3
> **Reps** 10

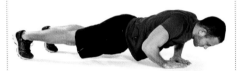

> **Form guide** p83

6 Weighted corkscrew
> **Sets** 3 > **Reps** 10

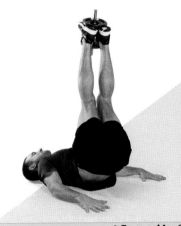

> **Form guide** p90

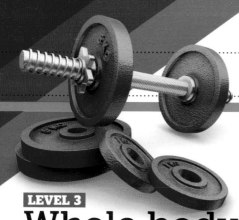

Do this ⬂

- **Do exercises 1-6 in order**
- **Rest for 1 minute between sets**
- **Rest for 2 minutes between exercises**

1 Turkish get-up
> **Sets** 2 > **Reps** 10 each side

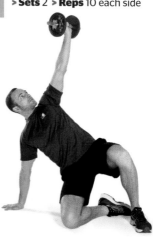

> **Form guide** p127

LEVEL 3

Whole-body
Workout

WHY DO IT?

Use challenging moves for your best ever body

This workout will be a challenge to anyone. You start with a technical whole-body move, the Turkish get-up, which is hard to master. Persevere, however, and the benefits will be worth it because it requires virtually every muscle in your body to go from lying to standing while holding a dumb-bell overhead.

The first move is followed by a testing lower-body move then a tricky upper-body move that also demands good core strength. You then repeat that pattern – doing a full-body move that involves a high level of co-ordination before doing a big lower-body move and a big upper-body move.

Snatch
> **Sets** 2
> **Reps** 10 each side

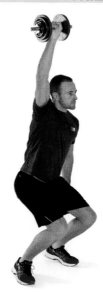

> **Form guide** p126

FIT TIP > Maintaining good form in the Turkish get-up and snatch is absolutely essential if you're to avoid injury and get the full benefit of these exercises.

2 Side lunge touch
> **Sets** 2 > **Reps** 10 each side

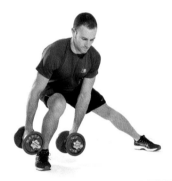

> **Form guide** p114

3 Press-up renegade row
> **Sets** 3 > **Reps** 10

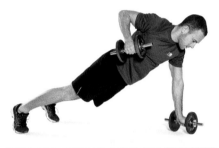

> **Form guide** p101

5 Jump squat
> **Sets** 3
> **Reps** 10

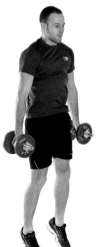

> **Form guide** p107

6 Rotating press
> **Sets** 2
> **Reps** 10 each side

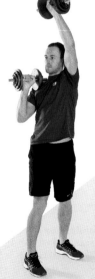

> **Form guide** p119

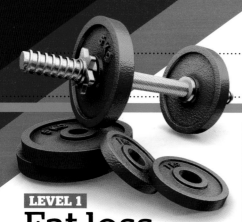

Do this ↘

- **Do 3 circuits**
- **Rest for 2 minutes between circuits**

1 **Dumb-bell press-up**
> **Time** 30 seconds

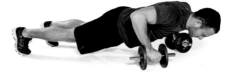

> **Form guide** p100

Fat loss
Circuit

WHY DO IT?

Burn calories and strip away fat

It's a common misconception that the best way to lose fat is to go for long runs. For anyone who doesn't enjoy plodding, the good news is that this is not the case. By far the best way of shifting unwanted weight is to do resistance circuits – a series of exercises performed back to back without rest.

This routine will work your entire body but it alternates between upper- and lower-body moves so while some muscle groups are working, others are resting. This allows you to work out at a high intensity, which raises your heart rate and burns more calories. Exercising like this will also fire up your metabolism so that your body keeps burning fat even after your workout.

4 **Lunge**
> **Time** 30 seconds
(alternate sides each rep)

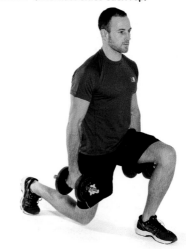

> **Form guide** p112

FIT TIP > Do as many reps as you can in the allocated time but don't be tempted to scrimp on form just to complete more reps.

Sumo squat
> **Time** 30 seconds

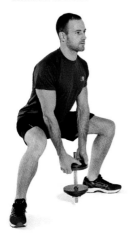

> **Form guide** p107

Bent-over flye
> **Time** 30 seconds

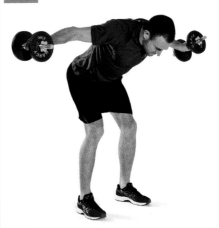

> **Form guide** p98

Curl to press
> **Time**
30 seconds

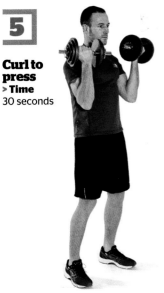

> **Form guide** p83

Rollout
> **Time** 30 seconds

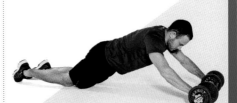

> **Form guide** p93

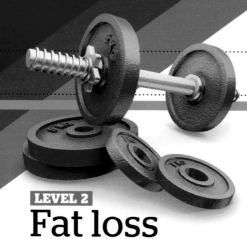

- **Do 3 circuits**
- **Rest for 2 minutes between circuits**

LEVEL 2
Fat loss
Circuit

WHY DO IT?

Build cardio fitness and get lean

The level two workout uses the same principles but this time the exercises are a bit more challenging. You still alternate between upper- and lower-body exercises but because the moves are more challenging your heart and lungs will have to work harder.

1
T press-up
> **Time** 30 seconds
(alternate sides each rep)

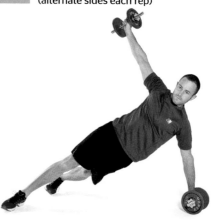

> **Form guide** p101

4
Side lunge
> **Time** 30 seconds
(alternate sides each rep)

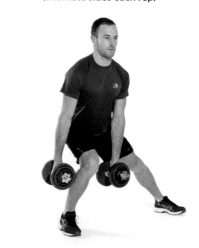

> **Form guide** p113

FIT TIP > If you have plate-loaded dumb-bells you won't have time to adjust the weight between exercises so choose a weight that allows you to complete the time in the most difficult exercise.

Squat
> **Time** 30 seconds

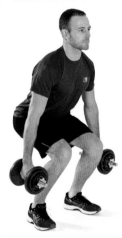

> **Form guide** p106

Upright row to shrug
> **Time**
30 seconds

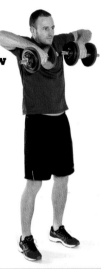

> **Form guide** p97

Alternating hammer curl with twist
> **Time**
30 seconds
(alternate sides
each rep)

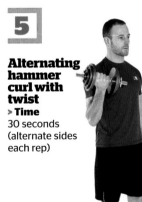

> **Form guide** p84

Alternating wide shoulder press
> **Time**
30 seconds
(alternate sides
each rep)

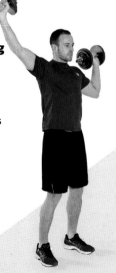

> **Form guide** p118

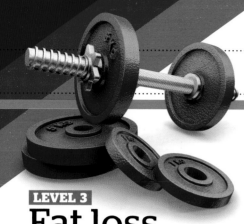

LEVEL 3
Fat loss
Circuit

WHY DO IT?

Challenge every body part and ditch your gut

This workout is an incredibly effective fat burner but it's also very demanding. You start with two intense explosive power moves that will really get your target muscles burning. After that it doesn't get any easier, with an unstable row, big hamstring move and a combination move to finish. You'll probably feel like the rest time between circuits is one minute rather than two.

1 **Ballistic press-up**
> **Time** 30 seconds

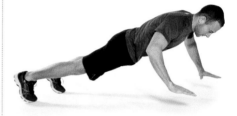

> **Form guide** p105

4 **Romanian deadlift**
> **Time** 30 seconds

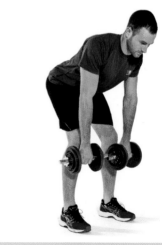

> **Form guide** p110

FIT TIP > The moves in this workout have been chosen because they should all allow you to lift a heavy weight. Choose the heaviest weight you can manage without compromising your form.

2

Jump squat
> **Time** 30 seconds

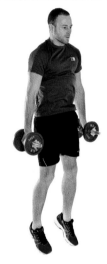

> **Form guide** p107

3

One-leg alternating bent-over row
> **Time** 30 seconds
(alternate sides after 15 seconds)

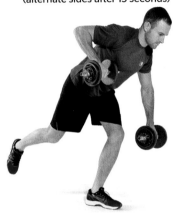

> **Form guide** p95

5

Zottman curl
> **Time** 30 seconds

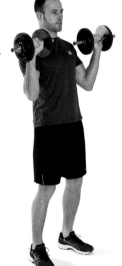

> **Form guide** p83

6

Lunge to press
> **Time** 30 seconds
(alternate sides with each rep)

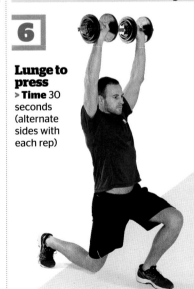

> **Form guide** p115

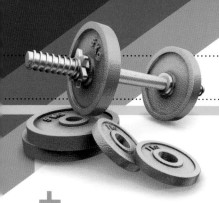

Total-body plan
Part 1

Weeks 1-4 Laying the foundations

There's a good reason why this part of the plan is called 'laying the foundations'. It's because it's the fundamental groundwork that you have to do if you eventually want to build lean muscle.

The exercises have been chosen because they encourage you to learn good movement patterns while also challenging your core strength. This means that when you come to increase the weight, your body will be able to respond positively to the increased stimulus. If you were tempted to skip this section, you wouldn't get the full benefit of the subsequent heavier weight weeks.

It's important to use light weights in this part of the plan so you don't overload your nervous system. You'll also notice that the set counts are relatively low and the rep counts are relatively high. This combination allows you to learn key movement patterns without overstressing your body.

Each workout targets your whole body. Every major muscle group is worked in at least one move, meaning that you hit every area three times a week. Stick to the plan and you'll be able to lift the heavier weights in weeks five to eight safely and confidently.

How to do the workouts

Timing
Do workouts A, B and C once a week each for four weeks, leaving at least one day's rest between workouts.

Weights
Use light weights for the exercises in these workouts. You should be able to complete each rep with perfect form. The aim of this month is to teach good movement patterns so you can increase the weight you lift in month two.

Tempo
Take one second to lift the weight, pause then take three seconds to lower the weight.

Sets and reps
The set counts in this phase are comparatively low, to allow you to complete the workouts. The rep counts, on the other hand, are comparatively high in order to build muscle endurance.

Rest periods
Rest for 45 seconds to one minute between sets and for 90 seconds to two minutes between exercises.

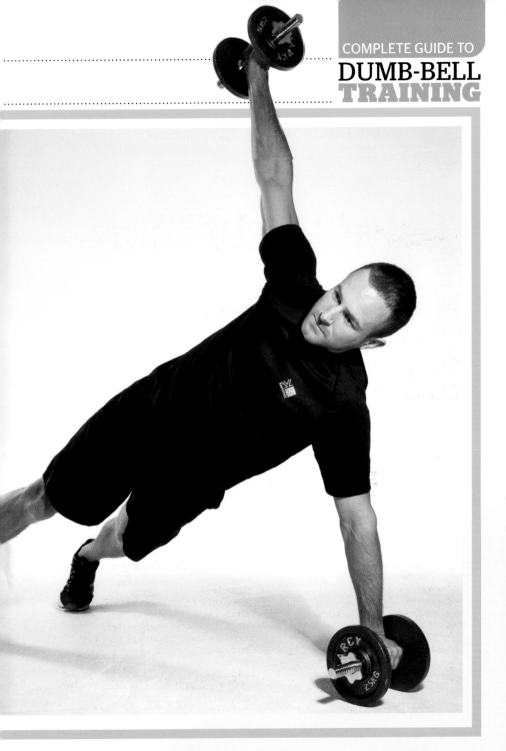

Weeks 1-4 Workout A

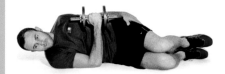

1 Internal rotations
> **Sets** 2 > **Reps** 12-15

2 External rotations
> **Sets** 2 > **Reps** 12-15

> **Form guide** p123

> **Form guide** p123

3 Woodchop lunge
> **Sets** 2 > **Reps** 12 each side

4 Step-up
> **Sets** 2 > **Reps** 12 each side

> **Form guide** p129

> **Form guide** p116

Press-up
> **Sets** 2 > **Reps** 12

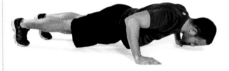

> **Form guide** p104

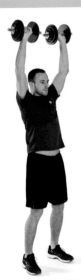

Shoulder press
> **Sets** 2
> **Reps** 12

> **Form guide** p117

Bent-over row
> **Sets** 2 > **Reps** 12

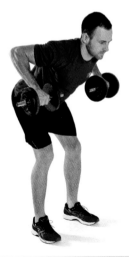

> **Form guide** p94

Dumb-bell rollout
> **Sets** 2 > **Reps** 12

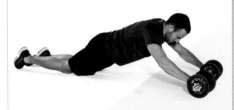

> **Form guide** p93

Weeks 1-4 Workout B

1

Woodchop
> **Sets** 2
> **Reps** 12
each side

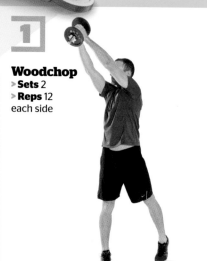

> **Form guide** p128

2

Dumb-bell press-up
> **Sets** 2 > **Reps** 12

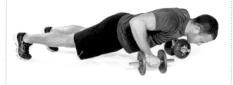

> **Form guide** p100

Side step-up
> **Sets** 2
> **Reps** 12
each side

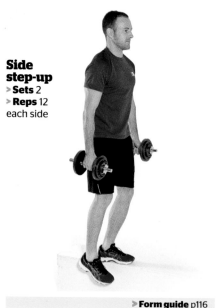

> **Form guide** p116

4

Renegade row
> **Sets** 2 > **Reps** 10 each side

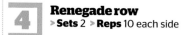
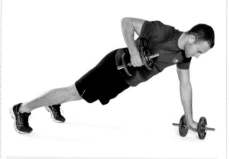

> **Form guide** p99

5. Side lunge touch
> **Sets** 2 > **Reps** 12 each side

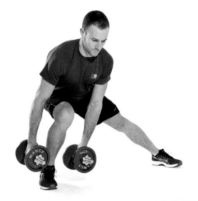

> **Form guide** p114

6. Cuban press
> **Sets** 2
> **Reps** 12

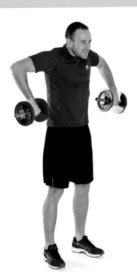

> **Form guide** p122

7. Dumb-bell squat
> **Sets** 2 > **Reps** 12

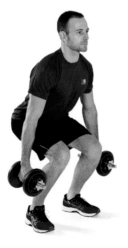

> **Form guide** p106

8. Side plank with lateral raise
> **Sets** 1 > **Time** 30 seconds each side

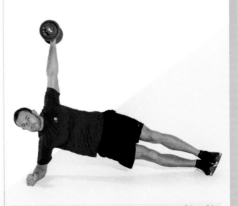

> **Form guide** p91

Weeks 1-4 Workout C

1

Diagonal lift
> **Sets** 2
> **Reps** 12 each side

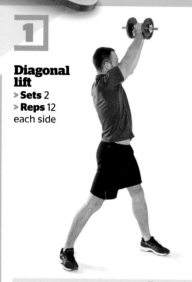

> **Form guide** p115

2 T press-up
> **Sets** 2 > **Reps** 8-10 each side

> **Form guide** p101

3 One-leg Romanian deadlift
> **Sets** 2 > **Reps** 12 each side

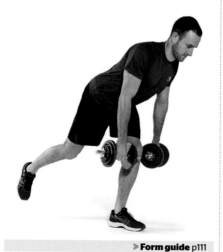

> **Form guide** p111

4 Around the world
> **Sets** 2
> **Reps** 12

> **Form guide** p124

5 Single-leg alternate bent-over row
> **Sets** 2 > **Reps** 12 each side

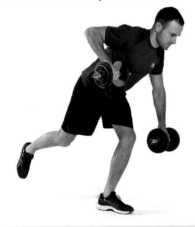

> **Form guide** p95

6 Trap three raise
> **Sets** 2 > **Reps** 12 each side

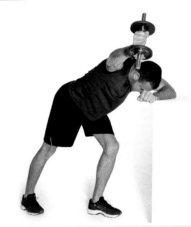

> **Form guide** p99

7 Bulgarian split squat
> **Sets** 2 > **Reps** 10-12 each side

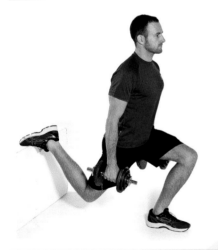

> **Form guide** p114

8 Seated Russian twist
> **Sets** 2 > **Reps** 12

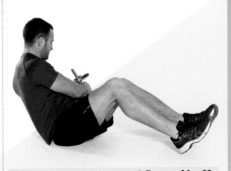

> **Form guide** p93

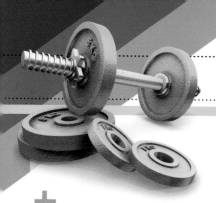

Total-body plan
Part 2

Weeks 5-8 Adding muscle

Now is the time when you can take advantage of all the good groundwork you did during the first four weeks. If you've been following the plan you will have instilled good movement patterns and you will have developed the stabilising muscles that you need to start lifting those heavy weights.

The workouts in this month are all based around big compound moves that work multiple muscle groups. Doing this type of move, as opposed to smaller isolation exercises that only target one muscle group, will elicit a bigger growth hormone release.

In the previous phase, lifting heavy weights wasn't important because all the focus was on establishing good movement patterns. In this phase you should aim to lift as heavy a weight as possible while maintaining perfect form.

How to do the workouts

Timing
Do workouts D, E and F once a week each for four weeks, leaving at least one day's rest between workouts.

Weights
You should use the heaviest weights you can manage to lift all the required reps. If you have to compromise your form to complete a rep, the weight is too heavy.

Tempo
Take one second to lift the weight, pause then take three seconds to lower the weight.

Sets and reps
The set and rep counts in this phase have been selected to give maximum hypertrophy (muscle growth) benefits.

Rest periods
Rest for one minute between sets and for two minutes between exercises.

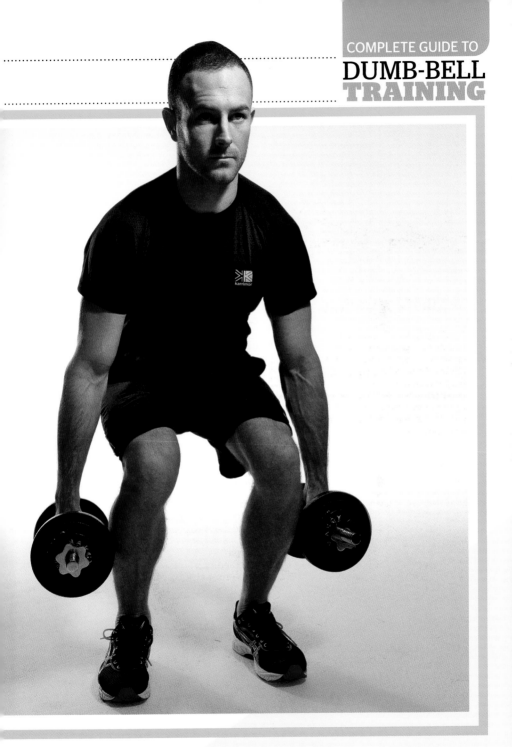

Weeks 5-8 Workout D

1
Lunge to press
> **Sets** 2 > **Reps** 8-10 each side

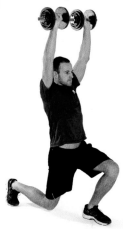

> **Form guide** p115

2
Dumb-bell floor press
> **Sets** 3 > **Reps** 8-10

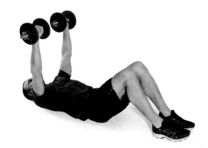

> **Form guide** p102

3
Reverse-grip bent-over row
> **Sets** 3 > **Reps** 8-10

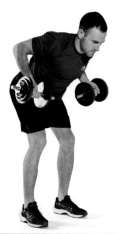

> **Form guide** p95

4
Sumo squat
> **Sets** 3 > **Reps** 8-10

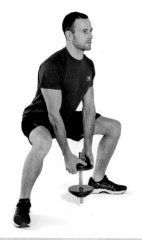

> **Form guide** p107

Shoulder press
> **Sets** 3
> **Reps** 8-10

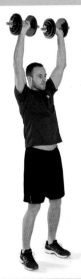

> **Form guide** p117

Biceps curl
> **Sets** 2 > **Reps** 8-10 each side

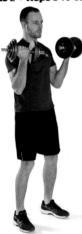

> **Form guide** p82

Overhead triceps extension
> **Sets** 2
> **Reps** 8-10 each side

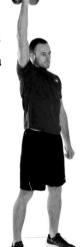

> **Form guide** p86

Dumb-bell crunch
> **Sets** 3
> **Reps** 8-10

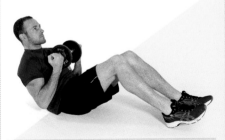

> **Form guide** p88

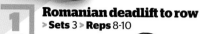

Weeks 5-8 Workout E

1 Romanian deadlift to row
> **Sets** 3 > **Reps** 8-10

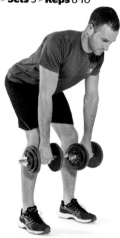

> **Form guide** p111

2 Diamond press-up
> **Sets** 3 > **Reps** 8-10

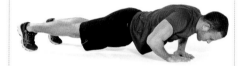

> **Form guide** p105

3 Upright row
> **Sets** 3
> **Reps** 8-10

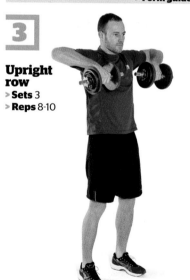

> **Form guide** p96

4 Lunge
> **Sets** 2 > **Reps** 8-10 each side

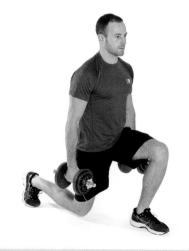

> **Form guide** p112

Push press
> **Sets** 3 > **Reps** 8-10

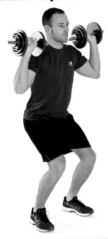

Hammer curl
> **Sets** 3
> **Reps** 8-10

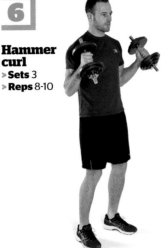

> **Form guide** 119

> **Form guide** p84

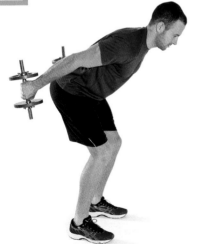

Two-arm kickback
> **Sets** 3 > **Reps** 8-10

Dumb-bell reverse crunch
> **Sets** 3 > **Reps** 8-10

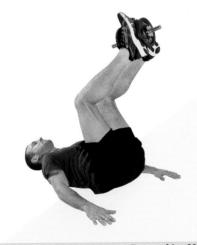

> **Form guide** p87

> **Form guide** p89

Weeks 5-8 **Workout F**

1

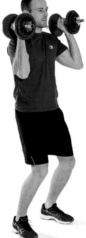

Hammer clean and press
> **Sets** 3
> **Reps** 8-10

> **Form guide** p125

2 **Press-up renegade row**
> **Sets** 2 > **Reps** 6-8 each side

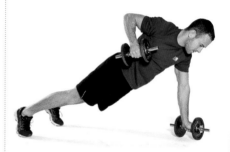

> **Form guide** p101

3 **Reverse lunge**
> **Sets** 2 > **Reps** 8-10 each side

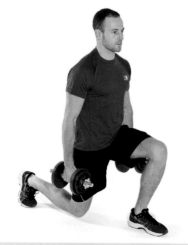

> **Form guide** p113

4

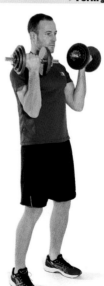

Arnold press
> **Sets** 3
> **Reps** 8-10

> **Form guide** p119

5 Romanian deadlift
> **Sets** 3 > **Reps** 8-10

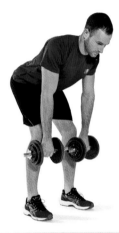

> **Form guide** p110

6 Zottman curl
> **Sets** 3
> **Reps** 8-10

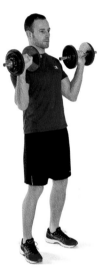

> **Form guide** p83

7 Overhead triceps extension
> **Sets** 2
> **Reps** 8-10 each side

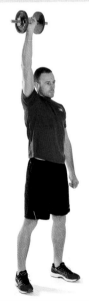

> **Form guide** p86

8 Dumb-bell side bend
> **Sets** 2 > **Reps** 8-10 each side

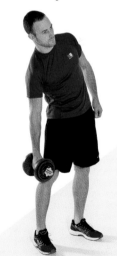

> **Form guide** p92

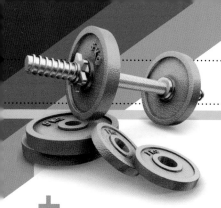

Total body plan
Part 3
Weeks 9-12 Stripping away fat

By this stage you should be looking bigger and feeling stronger. Now it's time to complete the plan by doing workouts that will strip away body fat, leaving you with lean, athletic-looking muscle.

The way you do that is by completing three full-body circuit workouts a week. This involves doing as many reps of a move as you can, with perfect form, for a particular amount of time before moving on to the next exercise. The moves in the workout alternate between upper- and lower-body moves, so you can go from one exercise to another with minimal rest. This means you keep your sessions intense, which helps you to melt away your body fat.

How to do the workouts

Timing
Do workouts G, H and I once a week each for four weeks, leaving at least one day's rest between workouts.

Weights
Choose a weight that you know you can handle for an intense workout. You get virtually no rest so your muscles will quickly become fatigued if you try to lift too heavy a weight.

Tempo
Do each rep as quickly as possible while maintaining perfect form. Don't scrimp on form to complete your reps swiftly.

Time
Do each exercise in order for the allocated time to complete one circuit.

Rest periods
Rest as little as possible between exercises and for two minutes between circuits. Aim to complete three circuits in total.

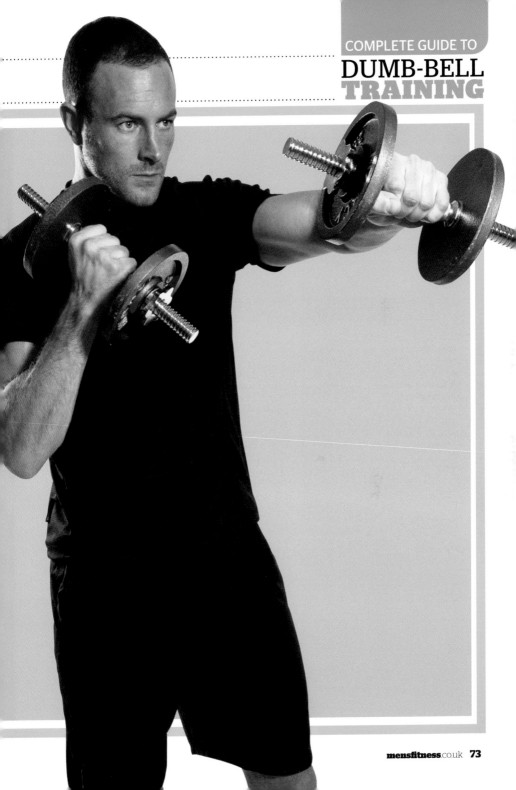

1 Turkish get-up
> **Time** 45 seconds

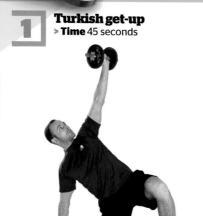

> **Form guide** p127

2 Ballistic press-up
> **Time** 45 seconds

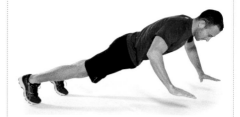

> **Form guide** p105

3 Bent-over flye
> **Time** 45 seconds

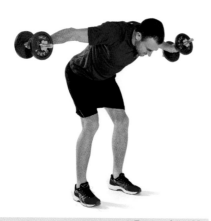

> **Form guide** p98

4 Side lunge
> **Time** 45 seconds

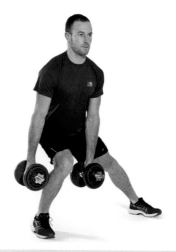

> **Form guide** p113

5 Curl to press
> **Time** 45 seconds

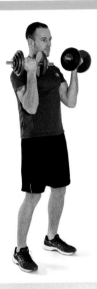

> **Form guide** p83

6 Rollout
> **Time** 45 seconds

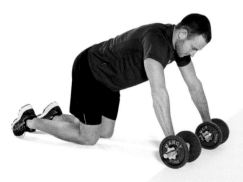

> **Form guide** p89

1

180° rotating woodchop
> **Time** 45 seconds

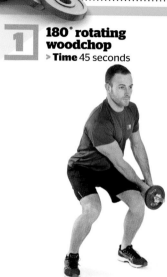

> **Form guide** p129

2

Upright row to shrug
> **Time** 45 seconds

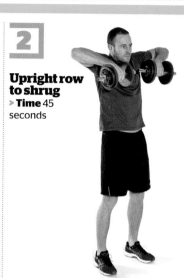

> **Form guide** p97

3

Jump squat
> **Time** 45 seconds

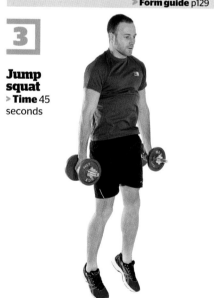

> **Form guide** p107

4

Halo
> **Time** 45 seconds

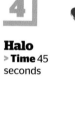
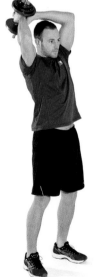

> **Form guide** p124

5 Side lunge touch
> **Time** 45 seconds

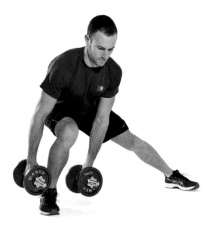

> **Form guide** p114

6 Dumb-bell uppercut
> **Time** 45 seconds

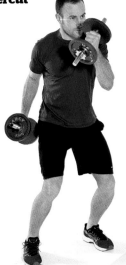

> **Form guide** p85

Weeks 9-12 Workout I

1 **One-arm snatch**
> **Time** 45 seconds

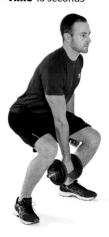

> **Form guide** p126

2 **T press-up**
> **Time** 45 seconds

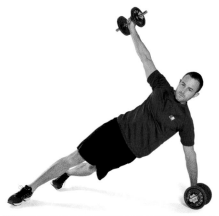

> **Form guide** p101

3

Side step-up
> **Time** 45 seconds

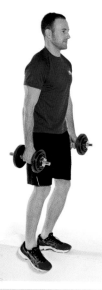

> **Form guide** p116

4 **Bent-over row**
> **Time** 45 seconds

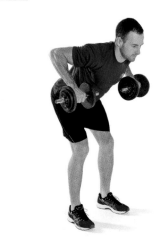

> **Form guide** p94

5 Squat to curl to press
> **Time** 45 seconds

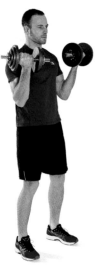

> **Form guide** p108

6 Dumb-bell punch
> **Time** 45 seconds

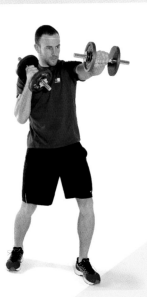

> **Form guide** p103

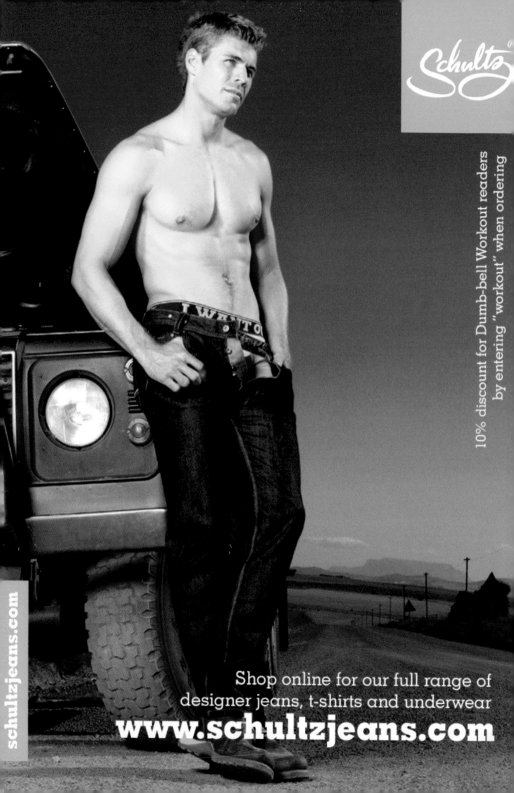

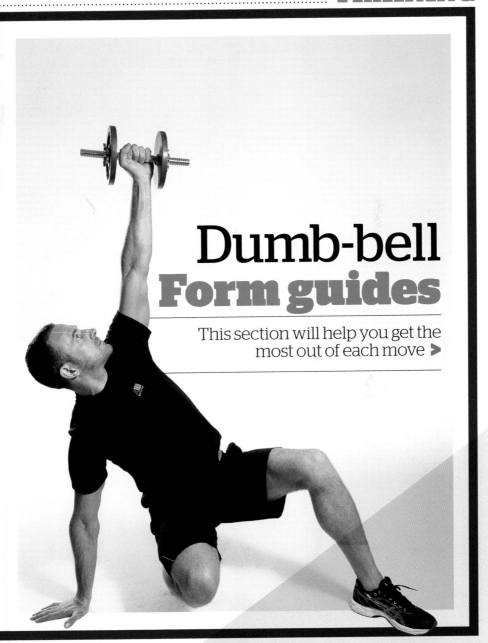

Dumb-bell
Form guides

This section will help you get the most out of each move >

Form Guides

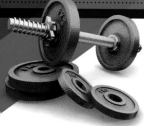

Biceps curl

● **Target** biceps
Using dumb-bells will work your biceps evenly, giving you balanced muscle growth.

> **Start position** With dumb-bells by your sides and arms facing forwards
● Keep your shoulders back and your core braced

> **Movement** As you lift the weights, keep elbows tucked into your sides and don't rock back and forth to use momentum
● Pause at the top of the move and lower slowly back to the start

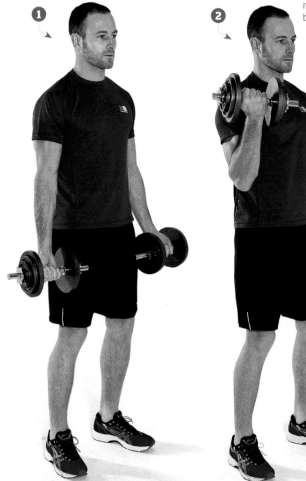

Concentration curl
● **Target** biceps
By locking your elbow in place you remove any upper-arm swing and focus the stress on your biceps.

> **Start position** Rest your elbow just inside your knee
> **Movement** Keep your upper body still and curl the dumb-bell up to your chest
● Rest your free hand on your opposite knee but don't press down on it to aid the move

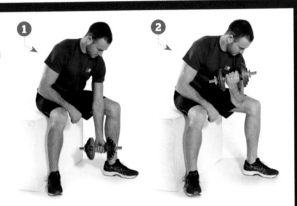

Zottman curl
● **Target** biceps
By rotating your wrists at the top of the move you transfer the emphasis on to your forearms for the lowering phase.

> **Start position** Dumb-bells by your sides and arms facing forwards
● Keep shoulders back and your core braced
> **Movement** As you lift the weight, keep your elbows tucked into your sides and don't rock back and forth to use momentum
● Pause at the top of the move and lower slowly back to the start

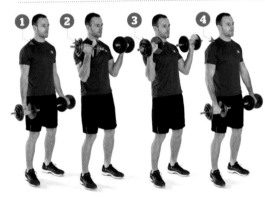

Curl to press
● **Target** biceps, shoulders
Combining a biceps curl with a shoulder press will give you a double muscle hit.

> **Start position** Dumb-bells by your sides and arms facing forwards
● Keep your shoulders back and your core braced
> **Movement** As you lift the weight, keep your elbows tucked into your sides and don't rock back and forth to use momentum

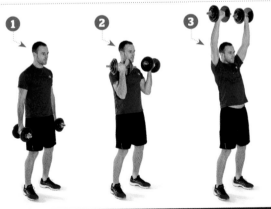

Form
Guides

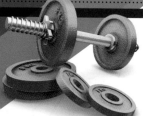

Hammer curl
● **Target** biceps
Curling the weight with a neutral grip takes some of the emphasis off your biceps and places more stress on your forearms.

> **Start position** Stand with your back straight, your shoulders back and your core braced
● Grip the dumb-bells with palms facing inwards and tuck your elbows into your sides
> **Movement** Curl the weight without rotating your wrists and make sure you keep your elbows tucked in
● Avoid rocking back and forth because this will allow you to use momentum to complete the movement

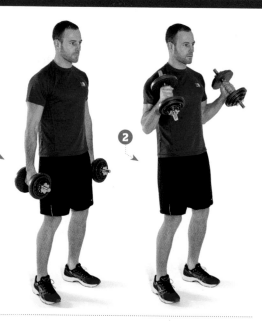

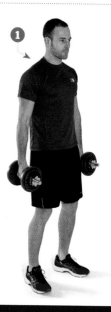
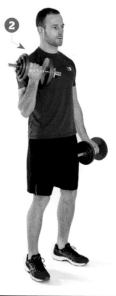

Hammer curl with twist
● **Target** biceps
Performing the move one arm at a time encourages you to stay upright and takes momentum out of the move. By rotating your wrists at the top of the move, you target your biceps from two angles.

> **Start position** Stand with your back straight, shoulders back and your core braced
● Grip the dumb-bells with palms facing inwards and tuck your elbows into your sides
> **Movement** Curl one dumb-bell up at a time, turning your wrists out at the top of the move to place extra tension on your biceps

Uppercut

● **Target** biceps
Punch yourself to bigger biceps with this high-tempo move.

> **Start position** Hold the dumb-bells by your chest with your elbows bent at 90°

> **Movement** Throw alternate uppercuts, pushing through your heels as you throw the punches to give them extra power

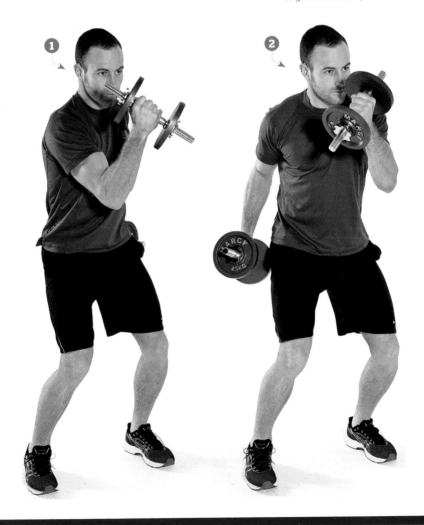

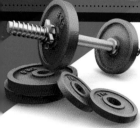

Overhead triceps extension

● **Target** triceps
This move encourages
you to stabilise your
body while working the
long head of the triceps
brachii for defined
looking muscles.

> **Start position** Stand
with your torso upright
and the weight above
your head with your arms
straight

> **Movement** Lower the
weight slowly by pivoting
at the elbow and keeping
your upper arm still
● Keep your body upright
throughout the move

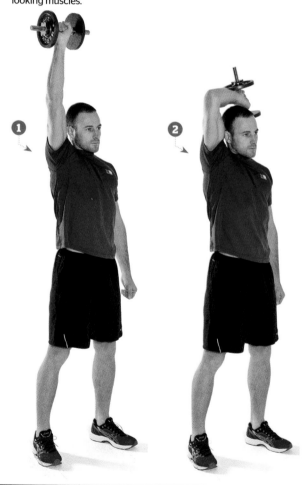

Two-arm kickback

● Target triceps, core
Work the triceps on both arms and challenge your core at the same time.

> Start position Bend forwards at the hips and keep your back in its natural arch
● Start with your elbows bent at 90°

> Movement Straighten your arms while keeping your upper arms as still as possible
● Keep your core braced throughout the move to maintain a neutral arch in your spine

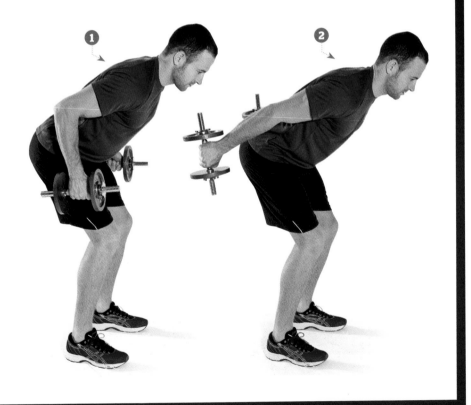

Form Guides

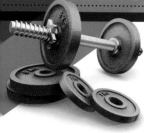

Crunch

● **Target** upper abs Adding weight rather than doing more reps will have a better muscle-building effect on your abs.

> **Start position** Keep both feet on the floor and your knees bent at 90° throughout the move
● Hold your head off the mat but keep your lower back in contact with the mat
● Hold the dumb-bell to your chest

> **Movement** Contract your abs to lift your shoulders off the mat, pause at the top of the move to squeeze your abs and slowly lower to the start

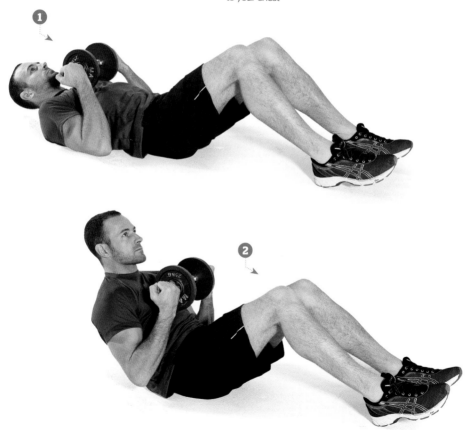

Reverse crunch

● **Target** lower abs
Your lower abs are
often neglected in
favour of doing upper
abs moves, such as
the crunch, but doing
this will help you get a
six-pack.

> **Start position** Lie
on the floor with your
feet flat on the floor and
your knees bent at 90°
● Hold a dumb-bell
between your feet

> **Movement** Keeping
your back on the floor,
contract your abs to
raise your hips off the
floor and lift the dumb-
bell up while keeping
your knees bent

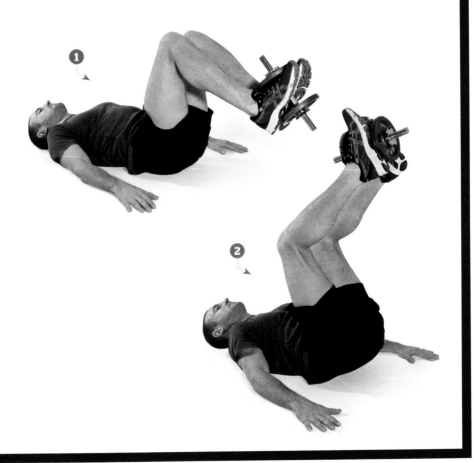

Form Guides

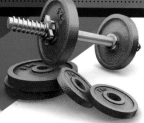

Weighted hip raise

● **Target** lower abs
The added weight makes this lower abs move a difficult but effective one.

> **Start position** Lie on your back with your legs in the air and your arms out to the side for balance
● Hold a dumb-bell between your feet

> **Movement** Lift your hips off the floor and push your feet towards the ceiling
● Hold for a second then slowly lower to the start

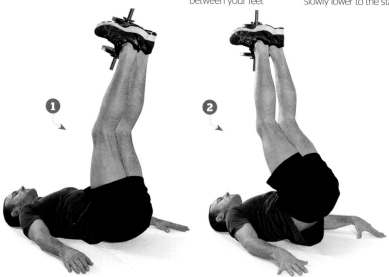

Weighted corkscrew

● **Target** lower abs
The two movements in this exercise give your lower abs a double hit. It's tough but it'll make them a lot stronger.

> **Start position** Lie on your back with your legs straight up in the air and your arms out to the side for balance.
● Hold a dumb-bell between your feet
> **Movement** Lift your hips off the floor and push your feet towards the ceiling
● At the top twist to one side, lower then repeat by twisting to the other side

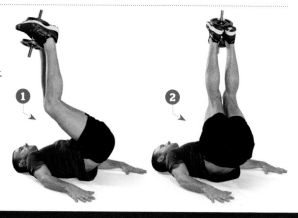

Side plank with lateral raise

● **Target** core, deltoids
Adding a lateral raise to a side plank increases the challenge to your core and improves your co-ordination.

> **Start position** Hold your body in a straight line from head to heels and position your elbow directly under your shoulder

> **Movement** Hold the plank position while slowly raising and lowering the weight
● Use a light weight to maintain perfect form

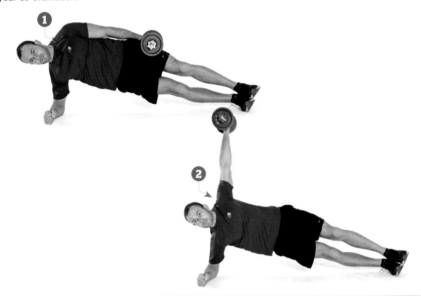

Side plank snatch

● **Target** core, obliques, shoulder
Moving the dumb-bell from a side plank position requires high levels of core control and co-ordination.

> **Start position** Get into a side plank position, as above
● Let the dumb-bell hang down across your stomach
> **Movement** Initiate the movement from your shoulder so you generate momentum that lifts the dumb-bell vertically until your arm is straight and pointing up

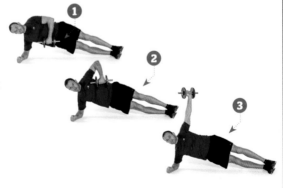

Form
Guides

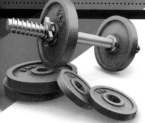

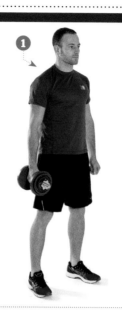

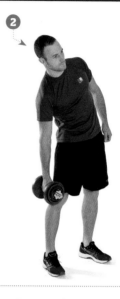

Side bend
● **Target** obliques
Use a heavy weight to really hit your
side abs in this standing move.

> **Start position** Hold a dumb-bell in
one hand by your side
> **Movement** Lean to the side holding
the dumb-bell then move as far as you
can to the other side without leaning
either forwards or backwards

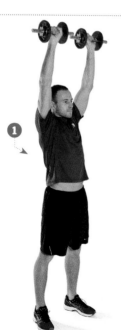

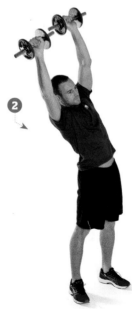

Saxon side bend
● **Target** obliques
Use light dumb-bells for
this move because your
outstretched arms create
long levers that your body
will struggle to control.

> **Start position** Stand
holding a dumb-bell in each
hand with your arms above
your head
> **Movement** Without
leaning forwards, bend your
torso to one side then return
to the middle

Seated Russian twist

● **Target** obliques
Work your side abs and your core with this functional exercise that's good for sports involving twisting moves.

> **Start position** Keep your back straight, your body at 45° to the floor and your knees bent at 45°
● Hold the dumb-bell in both hands in front of you
> **Movement** Twist your torso to one side but keep looking forward
● Twist your torso to the opposite side, using your abs to control the momentum

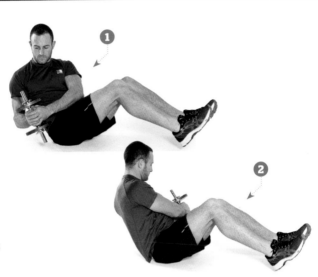

Rollout

● **Target** abs and core
This challenging move will build a rock-solid core but make sure you keep good form to prevent lower back injuries.

> **Start position** Kneel with your spine and neck neutral and your hands bellow your shoulders
> **Movement** Keeping your spine neutral, contract your abs to roll the dumb-bells out in front of you as far as you can without arching your back
● Roll the dumb-bells back to the start

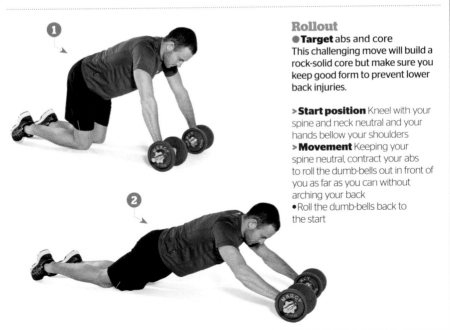

Form Guides

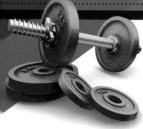

Bent-over row

● **Target** traps, lats, rhomboids
Doing this classic back-building move with dumb-bells will give you balanced muscle development because it prevents your stronger side form taking more of the strain.

> Start position Start with your back straight, your core braced and your shoulders retracted
● Lean forward from the hips, not the waist
● Stand with your feet shoulder width apart and bend your knees slightly
● Hold the dumb-bells just outside your knees

> Movement Pull the weights up to your sternum, allowing your wrists to turn naturally during the movement and squeeze your shoulder blades together at the top of the move
● Lower the dumb-bells slowly to the start

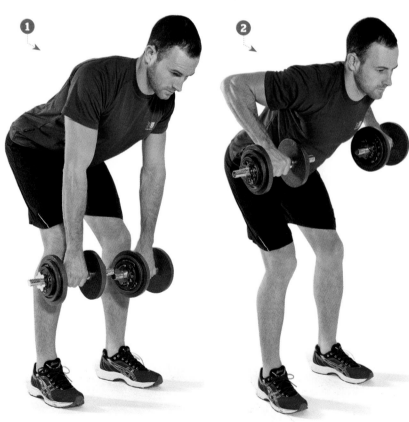

Reverse-grip bent-over row

● **Target** traps, lats, rhomboids, biceps
Reversing the grip on this classic move works your biceps as well as your back muscles.

> **Start position** Stand with your feet shoulder width apart, your back straight, your core braced and your shoulders retracted
● Lean forward from the hips, not the waist, and bend your knees slightly
● Hold the dumb-bells just outside your knees with your palms facing forwards
> **Movement** Pull the weights up to your sternum and squeeze your shoulder blades together at the top of the move
● Lower the dumb-bells slowly to the start

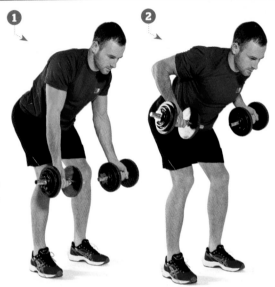

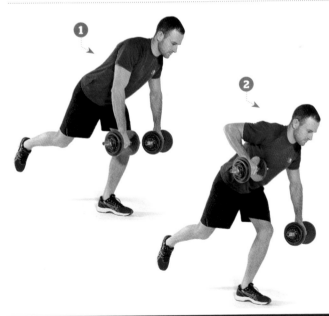

One-leg alternating bent-over row

● **Target** traps, lats, rhomboids, glutes, core
Doing the move on one leg recruits your glutes and calls on your core to stabilise your upper body.

> **Start position** Stand on one leg with your free leg behind you
● Lean forward from the hips, not the waist, and let the dumb-bells hang down either side of your standing knee
> **Movement** Alternately row one dumb-bell up to your body, keeping your body still

Form
Guides

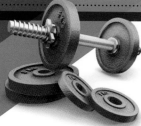

Upright row

● **Target** upper traps, shoulders
Develop your upper back and shoulders while increasing your upright pulling strength.

➤ **Start position** Hold the dumb-bells in front of your thighs

➤ **Movement** Raise your elbows to the sides to lift the dumb-bells up to your chest

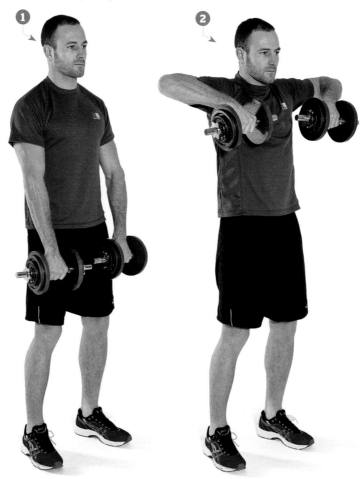

Shrug

● **Target** upper traps
Add size to your upper
back with this balanced
move, which will also help
stabilise your shoulder
girdle and reduce your
chances of sustaining a
shoulder injury.

> **Start position** Hold the
dumb-bells to your sides
with your palms facing
inwards and your shoulder
blades retracted
> **Movement** Raise
your shoulders straight
up without bending
your elbows and hold
the top position for one

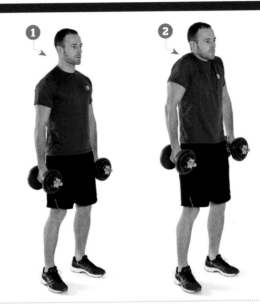

Upright row to shrug

● **Target** upper
traps, shoulders
Build impressive-
looking traps with
this double-hit
upper back move.

> **Start position**
Start with the
dumb-bells in front
of your thighs
> **Movement**
Raise your elbows
to the sides to lift
the dumb-bells up
to your chest
● Raise your
shoulders straight
up and hold the top
position for one or
two seconds

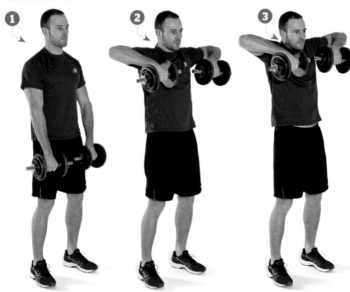

Form
Guides

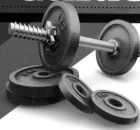

Bent-over flye

● **Target** upper back, shoulders
Get a strong upper back with this move that develops scapular retraction (the action of pulling your shoulder blades together).

> **Start position** Stand with your feet shoulder width apart, your back straight, your core braced and your shoulders retracted
● Lean forward, from the hips not the waist, and bend your knees slightly
● Hold the dumb-bells together just in front of your knees and keep a slight bend in your elbows

> **Movement** Raise the weights straight out to the sides without moving your upper body

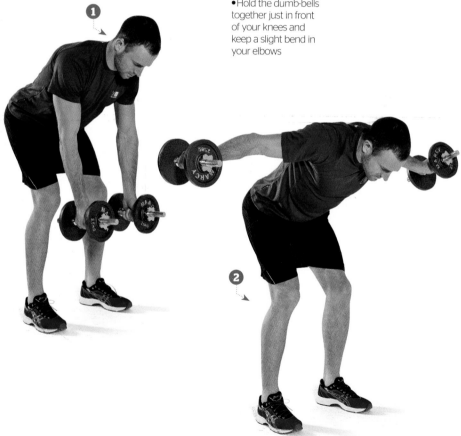

Renegade row
● **Target** lats, traps, rhomboids, core
Doing this impressive-looking move will challenge your core as well as your back because you have to stay strong in an unstable position.

> **Start position** Start by holding a pair of dumb-bells in the press-up position with your body straight from head to heels
> **Movement** Engage your core and row one of the dumb-bells up to your chest
● Return the dumb-bell to the start and repeat on the opposite side

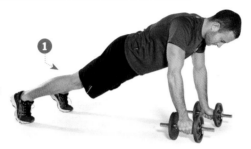

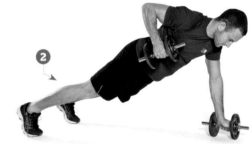

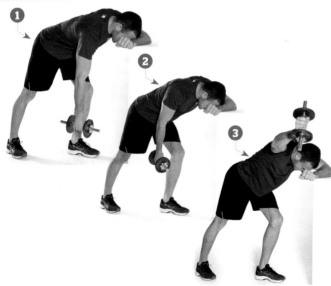

Trap three raise
● **Target** traps
Doing this move will improve your bench press because you'll be pressing from a more stable position. Make sure you use a very light weight.

> **Start position** Lean on a table for support and let a dumb-bell hang down by your shoulder
> **Movement** Retract your shoulder blade by pulling your shoulder back and down
● Lift the weight straight up and out to the side slightly before reversing the movement

Form Guides

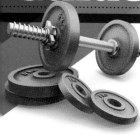

Dumb-bell press-up

● **Target** chest, triceps
Doing this classic move
while holding a pair of
dumb-bells will increase
the stability element of
the exercise.

> **Start position** Place
your hands level with your
shoulders, just wider than
shoulder width apart
● Keep your body in
a straight line from your
head to your heels
throughout the move

> **Movement** Lower
your body, making sure
you keep your elbows
pointing back rather than
to the sides

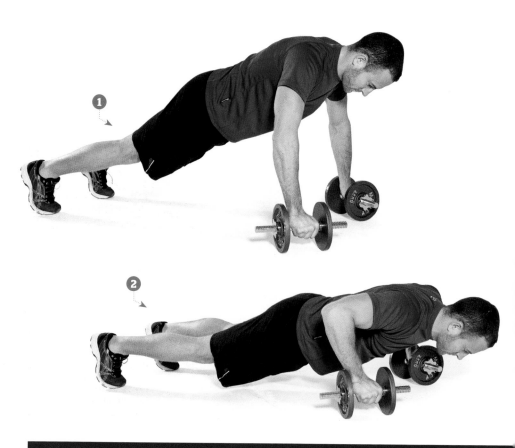

T press-up

● **Target** chest, shoulders, arms, core

Turn the press-up into an explosive move that works your body in more than one plane of motion.

> **Start position** Grip the dumb-bells with straight wrists and position them below your shoulders
• Keep your body in a straight line and your elbows tucked in
• Keep your feet shoulder width apart and don't let your hips sag
> **Movement** Push up powerfully and twist your body, rolling on to the sides of your feet and keeping your body in a straight line
• Raise a dumb-bell overhead with your arm straight then return to the start and perform the move on the opposite side

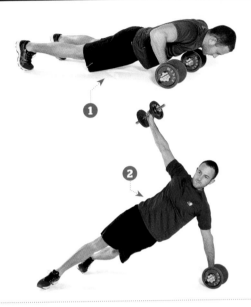

Press-up renegade row

● **Target** lats, traps, rhomboids, chest, core

Hit your back, chest and core with this demanding but satisfying move.

> **Start position** Start by holding a pair of dumb-bells in the press-up position with your body straight from your head to your heels
> **Movement** Perform a press up then row one of the dumb-bells up to your chest
• Return the dumb-bell to the start, perform another press-up then row the opposite dumb-bell up to your chest

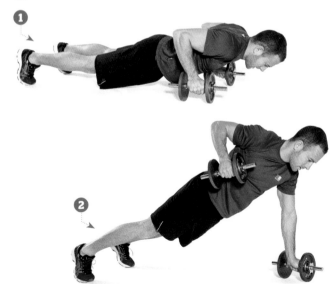

Form
Guides

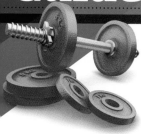

Floor press

● **Target** chest, triceps
Doing a press on the
floor lets you work
your chest muscles
with resistance, even
if you don't have a
bench or a gym ball

> Start position
Lie on your back with
your upper arms to the
sides on the floor and
your forearms vertical

> Movement
Bend your knees
and plant your feet
on the floor
● Press the dumb-bells
up amd then slowly
lower to the start

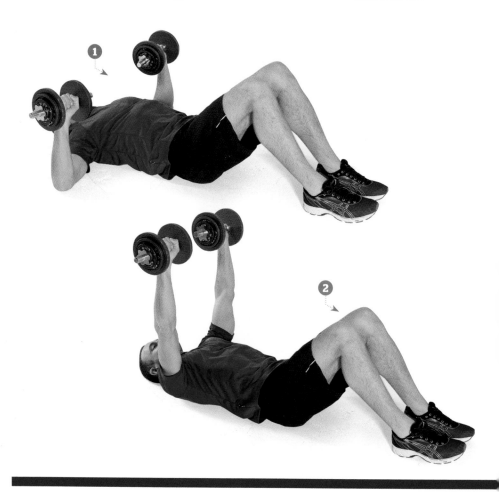

Punch

● **Target** chest, core, front shoulder
Throwing punches with dumb-bells will help build explosive power in your chest.

> **Start position**
Stand in a boxing stance while holding two dumb-bells
> **Movement** Throw alternate punches in a controlled and powerful movement

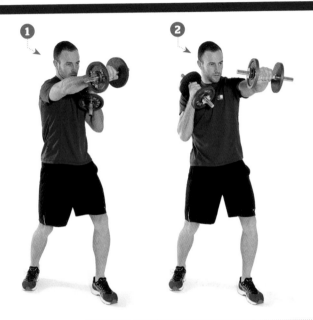

Hook

● **Target** chest
Use another boxing-inspired move to target your chest.

> **Start position** Stand in a boxing stance with low hands
> **Movement** Throw alternate hooks by swinging punches in a deliberate and powerful way across your chest

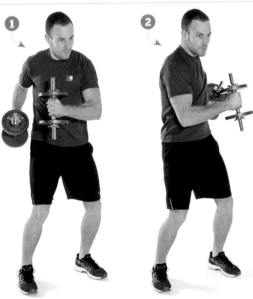

Form
Guides

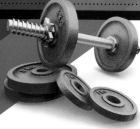

Press-up

Press-up
● **Target** chest, triceps
Do this classic move
to build your chest
and arms.

> Start position
Place your hands on
the floor level with your
shoulders, just wider than
shoulder width apart
● Keep your body in
a straight line from
head to heels throughout
the move

> Movement
Lower your body, making
sure you keep your
elbows pointing back
rather than to the sides

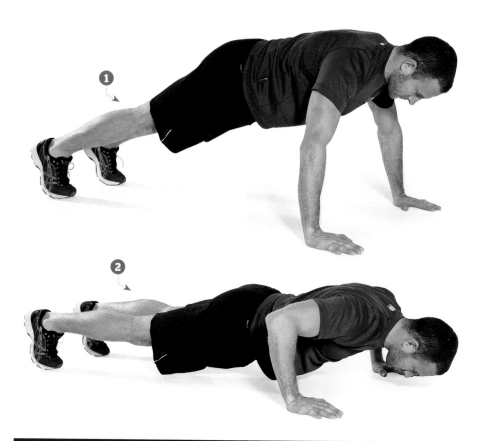

Ballistic press-up

● **Target** chest, triceps
Develop your fast-twitch
muscle fibres by pushing
up explosively so both
palms leave the floor.

> **Start position** Begin in
the press-up position
> **Movement** Lower
down, keeping your elbows
tucked in to your body
● Push up explosively so
your hands leave the floor,
land and go straight into
the next ballistic press-up

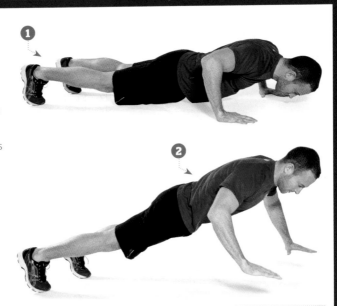

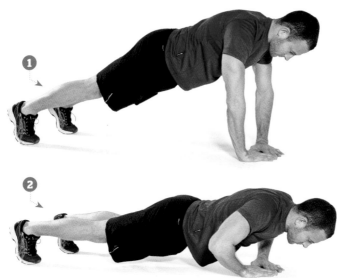

Diamond
press-up

● **Target** triceps,
chest
Placing your thumb
and index fingers
together shifts the
emphasis on to
your triceps.

> **Start position**
Hold your body in
a straight line from
your head to your
heels and your
thumbs and index
fingers together
so that they form
a diamond shape
> **Movement** Lower
your body, keeping
your elbows pointing
back rather than to
the sides

Form
Guides

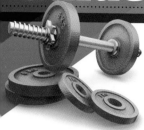

Squat

● **Target** quads, glutes, hamstrings
Hit several major muscle groups at once with this must-do leg move.

› Start position Stand with your feel shoulder width apart, your toes turned out slightly and your core muscles braced

› Movement Hold the dumb-bells by your sides and lower until your thighs are parallel with the ground
● Don't round your back and keep your knees in line with your feet
● Push back up through your heels

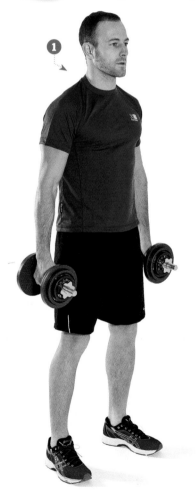

①

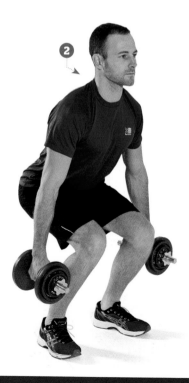

②

Jump squat

● **Target** quads, glutes, hamstrings
Turn the squat into a plyometric move and build explosive power.

> **Start position** Stand with your feel shoulder width apart, your toes turned out slightly and your core muscles braced
> **Movement** Hold the dumb-bells by your sides and lower until your thighs are parallel with the ground
● Don't round your back and keep your knees in line with your feet
● Push back up explosively through your heels so that your feet leave the ground
● Land and descend into another squat

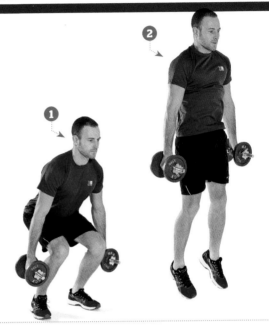

Sumo squat

● **Target** quads
By taking a wider stance you place more emphasis on the inside of your quads

> **Start position** Take a wide stance with your toes pointing out slightly
> **Movement** Grip a dumb-bell with both hands and lower until your thighs are parallel to the floor
● Keep your knees in line with your toes and keep your back upright

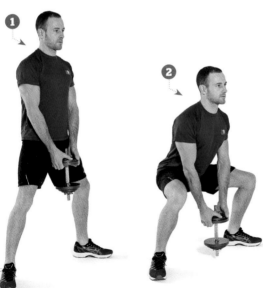

Form
Guides

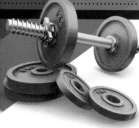

Squat to curl to press

● **Target** whole body
Put three exercises
together to make
one fluid move that
improves co-ordination
and works your whole
body without
overloading one joint.

> **Start position** Stand
with your feel shoulder

width apart, your toes
turned out slightly and
your core muscles braced

> **Movement** Sink into a
squat with your knees in
line with your feet
● As you stand up, curl
the dumb-bells up to your
shoulders, keeping your
elbows close to your sides

● Press the weights
directly overhead and
reverse the movement
back to the start

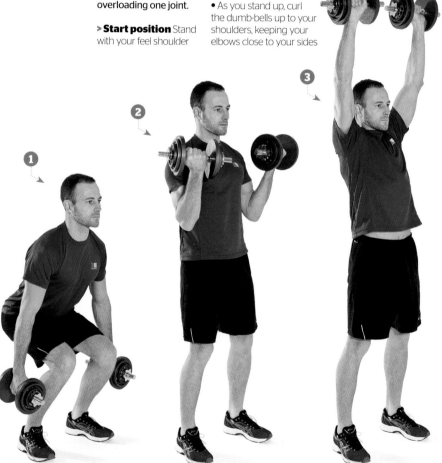

Rotating squat press

● **Target** whole body
Add a squat and rotation to turn a shoulder move into a whole-body exercise.

> **Start position** Hold the dumb-bells at shoulder level

> **Movement** Sink into a squat
● As you rise up, rotate your body and press the dumb-bell overhead, lifting your heel as you turn
● Return to the start and repeat the move on the other side

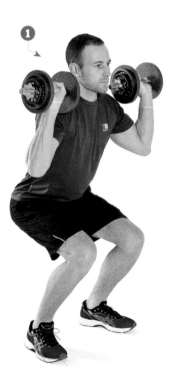

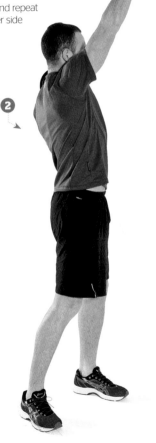

Form Guides

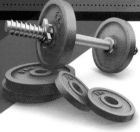

Romanian deadlift

● **Target** hamstrings
Develop the backs of
your legs but make sure
you use perfect form to
protect your back.

> **Start position** Start
in a split stance with the
whole of your front foot
and the toes of your back
foot on the floor

> **Movement** Hold
the weights either side
of your thigh and initiate
the move from your
hips, not your waist
● Keep your back flat
and let the weights travel
down your shins until you
feel a good stretch in your
hamstrings

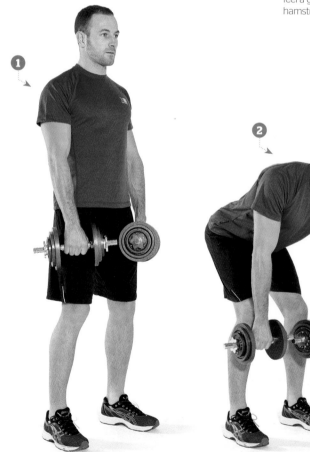

Romanian deadlift to row

● **Target** hamstrings, glutes, lats
Do this big combination move to work the posterior chain of your body.

> **Start position** Start by holding the dumb-bells by your thighs

> **Movement** Hold the weight either side of your thigh and initiate the move from your hips, not your waist

• Keep your back flat and let the weights travel down your shins until you feel a good stretch in your hamstrings
• Row the dumb-bells up to your sternum

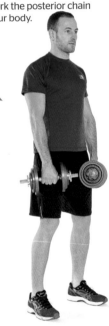
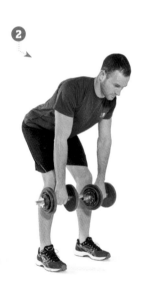
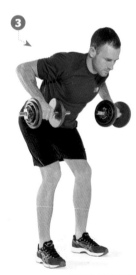

One-leg Romanian deadlift

● **Target** hamstrings
By standing on one leg you use your stabilising muscles and recruit your core to make sure you keep your balance.

> **Start position** Stand on one leg with your back foot raised and off the floor
> **Movement** Hold the weight either side of your thigh and initiate the move from your hips, not your waist
• Keep your back flat and let the weights travel down your shins until you feel a good stretch in your hamstrings

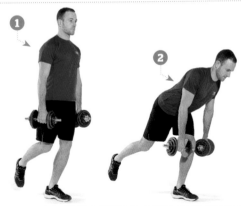

Form
Guides

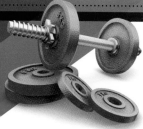

Dumb-bell lunge

● **Target** quads, hamstrings
Build muscle, increase your power and improve your co-ordination with this classic leg move.

> **Start position** Stand with your feet slightly apart, your back upright and the dumb-bells by your sides
> **Movement** Step forward and, in one fluid motion, bend your front knee and lower your

back knee until it almost touches the floor
● Keep your torso upright throughout the move and make sure your front knee is over your front toe
● Push off the front foot to return to the start

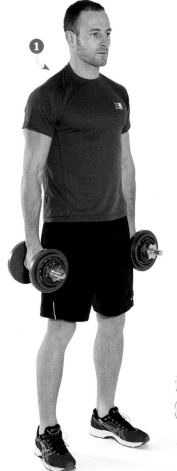

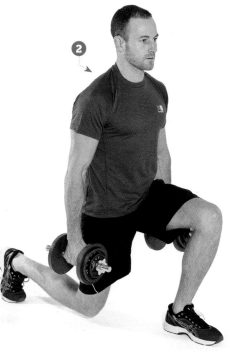

Side lunge
● **Target** adductors
Focus on your inner thighs to make sure you don't have any weak spots in your legs and improve your proprioception – the body's ability to sense it's movements.

> **Start position** Start with your feet close together and facing forward, your torso upright and dumb-bells by your sides
> **Movement** Take a big step to the side, lowering onto your leading leg
● Keep your torso upright throughout the move and your head facing forwards and your bent knee in line with your foot

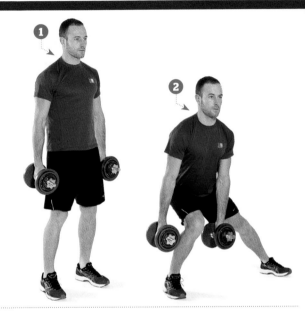

Reverse lunge
● **Target** quads, hamstrings
By stepping backwards instead of forwards you target your quads and hamstrings in a different way and increase the co-ordination challenge.

> **Start position** Stand with your feet slightly apart, your back upright and the dumb-bells by your sides
> **Movement** Step back into a lunge, bending your back leg so that your back knee nearly touches the floor
● Keep your torso upright throughout the move and make sure your front knee is over your front toe
● Push off the back foot to return to the start

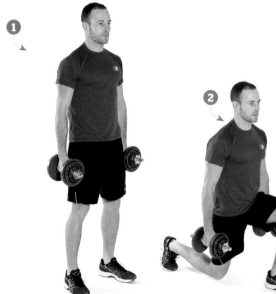

Form
Guides

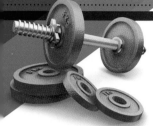

Side lunge touch
● **Target** quads, hamstrings, adductors
Work your hamstrings and quads, as well as your adductors with this progressive move.

> **Start position** Stand with your feet close together and facing forward, your torso upright and dumb-bells by your sides
> **Movement** Take a big step to the side, lowering onto your leading leg
● As you bend your leading knee, lower the dumb-bells until they touch either side of your foot

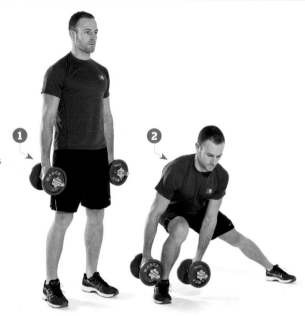

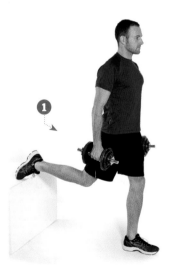

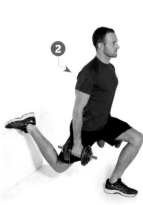

Bulgarian split squat
● **Target** quads, glutes
Placing one foot on the chair deactivates that leg and places all the emphasis on your front leg.

> **Start position** Rest the instep of your back foot on the chair and plant your front foot so it's facing forwards
● Your hips should be facing forwards and your torso should be upright with your core braced
> **Movement** Keeping your torso upright, lower until your front thigh is parallel to the floor
● Keep your front knee in line with your foot but make sure it doesn't travel beyond your toes

Lunge to press

● **Target** whole body
Combine two compound moves to challenge every major muscle group and improve your hip and lower back stability.

> Start position Stand with your feet apart, your back straight and the dumb-bells at shoulder height with your palms facing forward

> Movement Step forward into a lunge with your front knee over your front foot and your back knee close to the floor
● As you lunge forwards, press the weights directly overhead

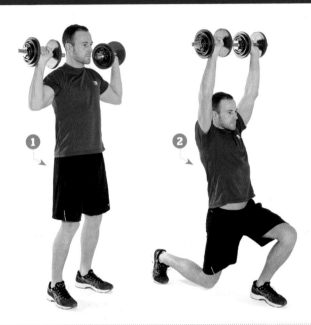

Diagonal lift

● **Target** quads, hamstrings, glutes, core, shoulders
This move hits multiple muscle groups at once and involves moving the weight through a full range of motion.

> Start position Start by holding a dumb-bell outside your bent knee with your trailing leg straight
> Movement Straighten your legs and simultaneously move the weights up and across your body, keeping your arms straight

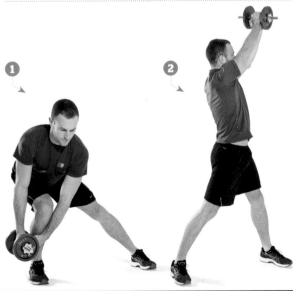

Form
Guides

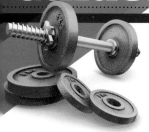

Step-up

● **Target** quads, glutes
This exercise has real-life benefits because you do this move every day when you climb stairs.

> **Start position** Try to find a chair or box that is no higher than knee height and place one foot flat on the top
● Keep your back upright and hold the dumb-bells by your sides
> **Movement** Push up with your leading leg while keeping your back upright
● Step back down with your trailing leg and repeat as before for all your reps before swapping sides

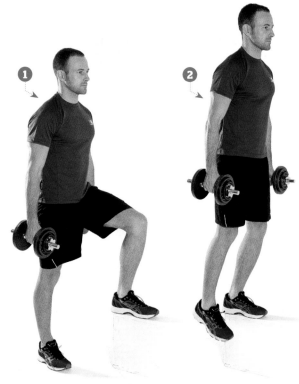

Side step-up

● **Target** quads, glutes
Work your legs and glutes form a different angle with this functional exercise.

> **Start position** Try to find a chair or box that is no higher than knee height and place one foot flat on the top with your other foot to the side
● Keep your back upright and hold the dumb-bells by your sides
> **Movement** Push up with your leading leg while keeping your back upright
● Step back down to the side with your trailing leg and repeat as before for all your reps before swapping sides

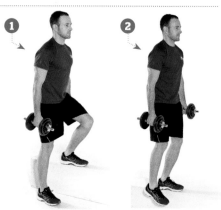

Shoulder press

● **Target** deltoids
Using dumb-bells allows your arms to move in a natural arc and will give you balanced muscle development.

> **Start position** Stand with your feet shoulder width apart and the dumb-bells held at shoulder height and your elbows out to the sides
• Keep your core braced throughout the move and avoid arching your back

> **Movement** Press the weights directly overhead but don't let the weights touch at the top

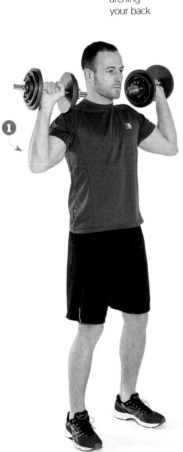

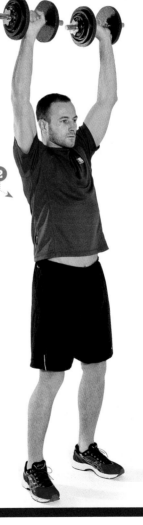

Form
Guides

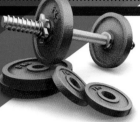

Seated shoulder press
● **Target** deltoids
Sitting down while doing the press makes the exercise more stable and allows you to lift more weight.

> **Start position**
Sit with your feet flat on the floor and the dumb-bells held at shoulder height and your elbows out to the sides
● Keep your core braced throughout the move and avoid arching your back
> **Movement** Press the weights directly overhead but don't let the weights touch at the top

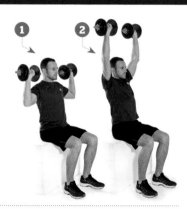

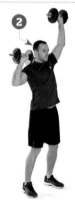

Alternating shoulder press
● **Target** deltoids
Focusing on one shoulder at a time makes each side work as hard as possible and gives you balanced muscle growth.

> **Start position** Stand with your feet shoulder width apart, your torso upright and your core braced
● Start with one dumb-bell at shoulder level with your elbow to the side and the other dumb-bell raised
> **Movement** As you lower one dumb-bell, raise the other, using your core muscles to stabilise the movement and avoid rocking

Alternating wide shoulder press
● **Target** deltoids
Hit your deltoids from a slightly different angle with this variation of the classic shoulder press.

> **Start position** Start with the dumb-bells at shoulder level
> **Movement** Press the weight at a 45° angle to your body
● You may need to use a slightly lighter weight than you would for a shoulder press

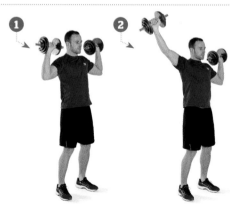

Arnold press
● **Target** deltoids
Introducing rotation to the move hits your deltoids from several angles in the same exercise.

> **Start position** Start with your palms facing you and your elbows out to the front.
> **Movement** Rotate your palms forward as you press the weights up
● End with palms facing forward and reverse the movement back to the start

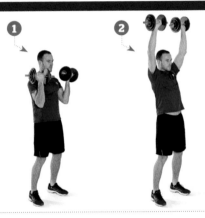

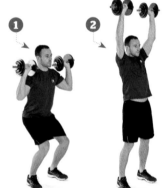

Push press
● **Target** shoulders
By using your legs to power the move you can lift a heavy weight and move explosively.

> **Start position** Stand with your feet shoulder width apart, the dumb-bells held at shoulder height and your elbows out to the sides
● Keep your core braced throughout the move and avoid arching your back
> **Movement** Sink down into a quarter squat then straighten your legs and simultaneously press the weights directly overhead but don't let the weights touch at the top

Rotating press
● **Target** shoulders
Adding a rotation to the press challenges your core stabilising muscles as well as your side abs.

> **Start position** Stand with your feet shoulder width apart and the dumb-bells held at shoulder height and your elbows out to the sides
> **Movement** Press one dumb-bell overhead and, as you do so, rotate your torso.

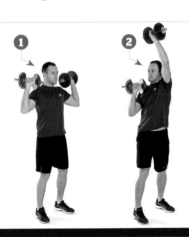

Form
Guides

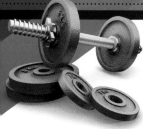

Lateral raise

● **Target** middle deltoid, traps
Use a light weight to target both your delts and your upper traps to give yourself broad-looking shoulders.

> **Start position** Stand with your feet shoulder width apart, your body upright and your core braced

> **Movement** Lift the weights out to the sides with straight arms
● Stop at shoulder level and hold for a moment before lowering slowly

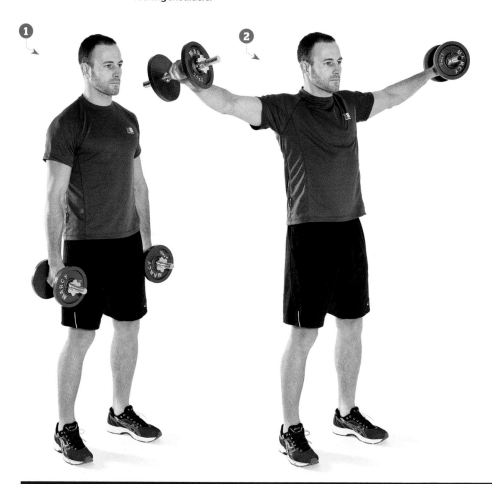

Front raise
● **Target** front deltoid
By raising the dumb-bells out in front of you, you place the stress on your front shoulders.

> **Start position** Hold the dumb-bells in front of your thighs with your palms facing you
> **Movement** Lift the dumb-bells out in front of you to shoulder level, pause and lower slowly to the start

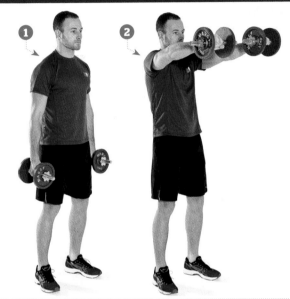

Front/lateral raise
● **Target** middle, front deltoids
Alternate between front and lateral raises each time you lift the weight to hit your front and middle deltoids in the same move.

> **Start position** Hold one dumb-bell by your side and the other in front of your thigh
> **Movement** Lift the weights to the front and to the side simultaneously, pause at the top before slowly lowering and swapping sides each rep

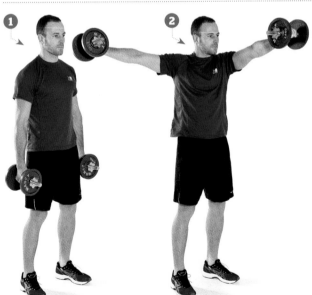

Form Guides

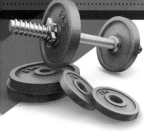

Cuban press

● **Target** rotator cuff
Strong and stable rotator
cuffs are vital if you want
to avoid shoulder injuries
during heavy lifts. This
move targets that often
neglected muscle.

> **Start position** Hold
the dumb-bells out to
your sides with your
arms straight and your
palms facing back

> **Movement** Lift
your arms out to the
sides until your elbows
are bent at 90 degrees
with the weights hanging
straight down
● Rotate your arms
so your hands point
up, keeping your upper
arms horizontal
● Press the weights
directly overhead and
reverse the movement
back to the start

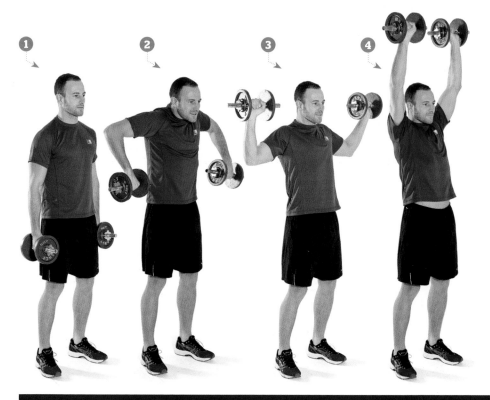

Internal rotation
● **Target** rotator cuff
Do this move as a warm-up before heavy shoulder exercises or at the end of a workout to develop your stabilising muscles.

> Start position Lie on your side with your knees bent for stability and your upper arm in line with your body and your elbow bent at 90°
● Hold a light dumb-bell with an upturned palm
> Movement Rotate your arm so the dumb-bell points upwards with your elbow still at 90°

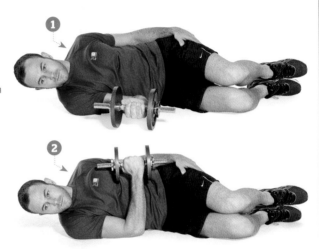

External rotation
● **Target** rotator cuff
Move your shoulder in the opposite direction to the internal rotation.

> Start position Lie on your side with your knees bent for stability
● Hold a dumb-bell with your upper arm in line with your body and your elbow bent at 90°
> Movement Rotate your arm as far as is comfortable and return to the start

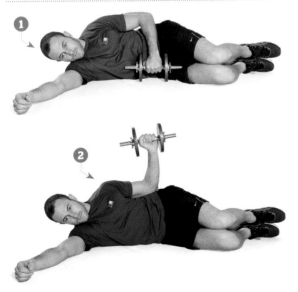

Form
Guides

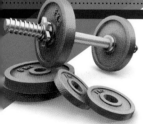

Halo
● **Target** shoulders
Moving the dumb-bell around your head in a 360° rotation works your whole shoulder joint.

> **Start position** Hold the dumb-bell in front of you at chin height.
> **Movement** Rotate the dumb-bell around your head then reverse the movement back to the start.

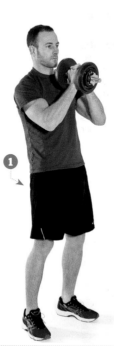

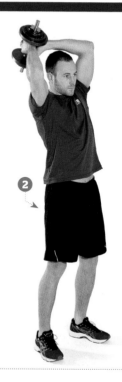

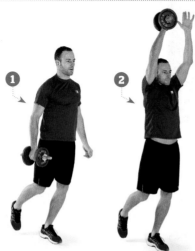

Around the world
● **Target** shoulders, core
Use a light dumb-bell for this deceptively difficult move, which targets your middle shoulder as well as your balance.

> **Start position** Stand on one leg and hold a dumb-bell in front of your thigh
> **Movement** Raise your hands up in and arc until both hands are above your head
● Swap the dumb-bell into your opposite hand and bring your arms down to your sides in an arc

Hammer clean and press

● **Target** hamstrings, glutes, calves, back, shoulders
This move is usually performed with a barbell but you can do it with dumb-bells to make sure that both sides of your body are working equally hard.

> **Start position** Stand with the dumb-bells by your sides
> **Movement** Sink into a quarter squat then straighten up and lift the dumb-bells up to shoulder height by using momentum and shrugging your shoulders and bending at your elbows

● Bend your knees slightly then straighten your arms to press the weights directly overhead

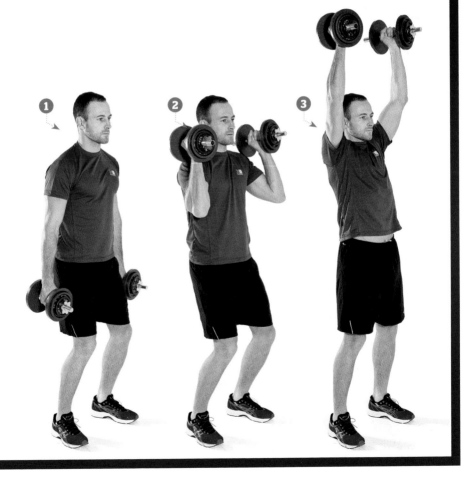

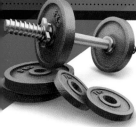

One-arm snatch

● **Target** whole body
This whole body move
requires considerable
co-ordination and
develops power so
it's great for sports
such as football and
rugby that require
you to generate force
in an upright position.

> **Start position** Start
with your knees bent
and hold one dumb-bell
between your
legs, keeping your
shoulders square on

> **Movement** Straighten
your legs and use the
momentum to lift the
weight up in front of
you powerfully
● Squat down beneath
the weight to catch it with
your arm straight
● Stand up straight to
complete the move

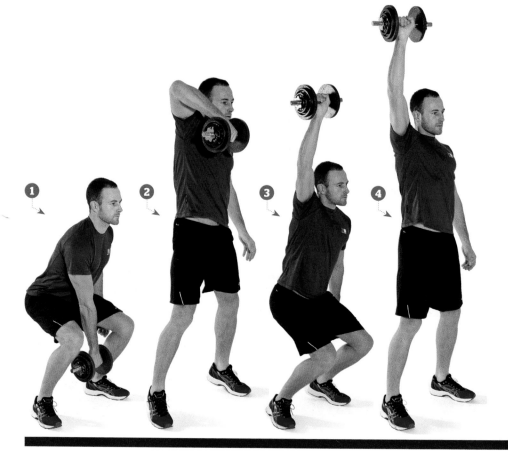

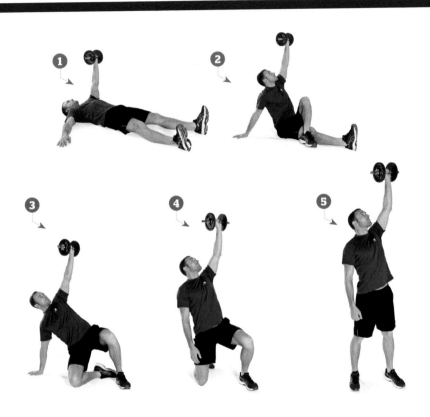

Turkish get-up

● Target whole body
Even when using a
comparatively light weight
this is a great all-over muscle
and co-ordination builder.

> Start position Lie flat on the
floor with one hand by your side
for balance and the other vertical
and holding a dumb-bell

> Movement Keeping your
non-working arm straight, start
to swing the leg in the dumb-bell
side over your opposite leg
● As you plant your foot, rise up
onto your elbow
● Extend your supporting arm
then move onto the knee of the
leg that's on the floor
● Take your supporting hand off
the floor, move your torso to an
upright position before standing
up with the dumb-bell overhead

Form
Guides

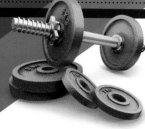

Woodchop

● **Target** whole body This move is great for sports like tennis that require twisting power because it connects your upper and lower body with one big rotational lift.

➤ **Start position** Stand with your feet shoulder width apart and your knees bent so that your thighs are almost parallel to the floor
• Keep your back flat and twist your torso to the side, holding a dumb-bell in both hands on the outside of your thigh

➤ **Movement** As you stand up, turn your torso to the opposite side, lifting the dumb-bell up and across your body with straight arms
• Use your core muscles to control the movement and pivot on your back foot as you twist

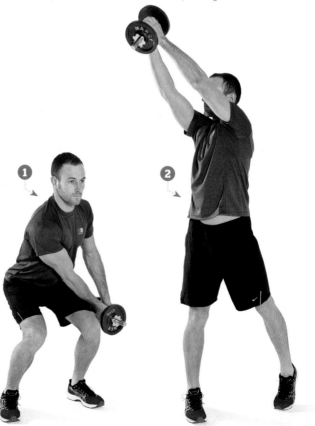

Woodchop lunge

● **Target** whole body
This move gets your body
moving across three
planes, which tests your
balance and co-ordination,
and makes it a great move
for sports conditioning.

> **Start position** Stand
up straight and hold a
dumb-bell in both hands
over one shoulder
> **Movement** Step forward
into the lunge and chop the
weight down and across
your body
• Make sure your front foot
faces forward, your front
knee is over your foot and
your back is straight

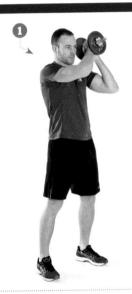
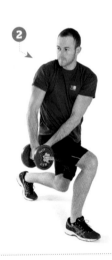

180° rotating woodchop

● **Target** Whole body
Make the woodchop explosive
by simultaneously jumping
and twisting. You need good
balance to control your
movement as you land.

> **Start position** Start with your
feet shoulder width apart and your
knees bent so that your thighs are
almost parallel to the floor
• Keep your back flat and twist
your torso to the side, holding a
dumb-bell in both hands on the
outside of your thigh

> **Movement** Move the weight
up and across your body and,
as you do so, jump up and
rotate 180°
• Your arms should be up and
above your shoulder as you pass
through 90°. You should lower
your arms across your body at
between 90 and 180°

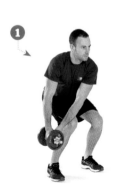
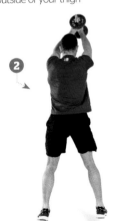
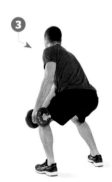

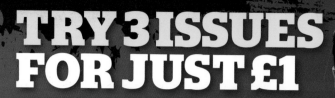
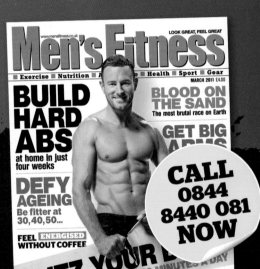
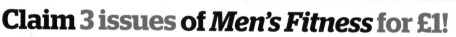